SOCIALIZATION GAMES FOR PERSONS WITH DISABILITIES

ABOUT THE AUTHORS

Nevalyn F. Nevil, M.A., L.P.C.C., is a clinician, consultant, and trainer for agencies serving persons with disabilities in and around Central Ohio. She is a managing associate of the Overbrook Clinic, Columbus, Ohio.

Marna L. Beatty, M.A., L.P.C.C., is a clinician and consultant to families and agencies serving persons with disabilities. She specializes in services to persons with behavioral challenges and is an associate of the Overbrook Clinic, Columbus, Ohio.

David P. Moxley, Ph.D., is an associate professor in the School of Social Work, Wayne State University, Detroit, Michigan.

SOCIALIZATION GAMES FOR PERSONS WITH DISABILITIES

Structured Group Activities for
Social and Interpersonal Development

By

NEVALYN F. NEVIL

MARNA L. BEATTY

DAVID P. MOXLEY

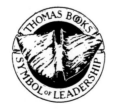

CHARLES C THOMAS • PUBLISHER, LTD.
Springfield • Illinois • U.S.A.

Published and Distributed Throughout the World by

CHARLES C THOMAS • PUBLISHER, LTD.
2600 South First Street
Springfield, Illinois 62794-9265

© *1997 by* CHARLES C THOMAS • PUBLISHER, LTD.

ISBN 0-398-06746-5 (paper)
ISBN 0-398-06749-X (cloth)

Library of Congress Catalog Card Number: 96-37683

With THOMAS BOOKS *careful attention is given to all details of manufacturing
and design. It is the Publisher's desire to present books that are satisfactory as to their
physical qualities and artistic possibilities and appropriate for their particular use.*
THOMAS BOOKS *will be true to those laws of quality that assure a good name
and good will.*

Printed in the United States of America
SC-R-3

Library of Congress Cataloging-in-Publication Data

Nevil, Nevalyn.
    Socialization games for persons with disabilities : structured
group activities for social and interpersonal development / by
Nevalyn F. Nevil, Marna L. Beatty, David P. Moxley.
        p.   cm.
    Includes bibliographical references and index.
    ISBN 0-398-06746-5 (pbk.)   ISBN 0-398-06749-X (cloth)
    1. Handicapped—Rehabilitation.   2. Socialization.   3. Social
skills—Study and teaching.   4. Educational games.   I. Beatty,
Marna L.   II. Moxley, David.
    HV1568.3.N49   1997
    616.85'8806—dc21
                                                                96-37683
                                                                CIP

PREFACE

The purpose of *Socialization Games for Persons with Disabilities* is to
provide professional and support personnel with a practical frame-
work for encouraging positive social behavior. Although the socialization game approach was conceived of as a technique for working on
institutional living areas for persons with mental retardation and severe
behavior problems, the approach has been used with different popula-
tions in an array of programmatic environments. Since the publication
of *Socialization Games for Mentally Retarded Adolescents and Adults (1980)*,
hundreds of games have been introduced for therapeutic use. Games
have been used effectively with children, adolescents and adults with a
range of functional abilities and limitations. Settings have included
vocational, rehabilitation, educational, residential and treatment programs.
Thus, teachers, social workers, counselors, psychologists, vocational and
rehabilitation specialists and recreation therapists, as well as direct support staff, will find this book relevant to the social development of
persons they serve.

The design of the book lends itself to the implementation of a socialization program. The first section introduces the socialization game approach.
It provides an overview of the development of our approach, then, a
rationale for the use of socialization games and a discussion of their
design. As our approach requires a group format, section two outlines
specific considerations one should take into account when forming a
group. The third section is devoted to group leadership. It focuses on
desirable characteristics of a group leader and examines the goals and
tasks of group leadership. The fourth section describes three types of
group programs designed to focus on basic social skill development,
work adjustment and conflict resolution. The last section includes a
game assessment scheme that analyzes, along several dimensions, over
100 socialization games that are presented in this section. The assessment
scheme will assist leaders in selecting games that are appropriate for
members of their particular group.

We want to emphasize that it is not our intention to provide readers with a packaged approach to a socialization program. We hope that our concepts and ideas will blend usefully with the reader's own creative ideas and plans. Through such collaboration, we can realize more innovative and practical ways of providing critical programming in the areas of socialization and social skill development.

ACKNOWLEDGMENTS

We gratefully acknowledge the significant contribution that numerous individuals have made to assist us with the completion of this revision. First and foremost, we would like to thank our mentor and friend, Barbara Edmonson, for her persistent encouragement and support of our efforts throughout the project. Barb revitalized the game approach and us in the process. We also wish to recognize our secretary, Barbara Lewis, who spent countless hours preparing and revising our manuscript drafts. Finally, we would like to express our sincere appreciation to the many individuals who have cooperated with and contributed to the development of our games. Beginning with the unique contributions of the game group at Forest Cottage and continuing with countless other participants in many different game programs, we have learned much about designing games that work. Feedback and suggestions for modifications from group members have been essential to the development of new games. We have also continued to be affirmed, by persons of all ages and abilities, that socialization games provide a fun and interesting approach to learning more about ourselves and developing positive relationships with others.

CONTENTS

SOCIALIZATION GAMES FOR PERSONS WITH DISABILITIES

SECTION 1

THE SOCIALIZATION GAME APPROACH

BACKGROUND

The socialization game approach evolved over a two-year period of work on two security areas of a state-operated developmental center for persons with mental retardation. Most of the thirty women who lived in these areas were functioning in the moderate range of mental retardation; others, in the severe range. Almost all of the women had adequate levels of self-care skills, but were characterized by high levels of aggressive and destructive behavior. Because of their severe difficulties in getting along with others they were, for the most part, excluded from programming and were confined to their living areas around the clock. Threats, insults, screaming, fighting, biting, and the destruction of property were frequent occurrences. Distrustful of interpersonal contact, many of the residents spent much of their time isolated in the corners of their living area or lying on their beds. Positive social interaction between the residents was rare. Occasions for positive group social interaction were seldomly provided.

Conditions on the living area contributed to the atomistic behavior. Many of the women had long histories of institutionalization characterized by deprivation, punishment and abuse. Overworked and undertrained aides lacked the motivation, knowledge, or the technical support to implement habilitative activities. A primary goal of the aides was to maintain control. They attempted this by keeping residents apart and isolated and by severe punishment for transgressions. A frequent punishment was to take a prized possession from a resident who may have broken a rule, or acted out. This would result in an outburst of rage, and a whole cycle of behavioral contagion would be set in motion. The punished resident would displace her anger onto someone lower in the pecking order and the displacement response would continue until virtually every resident was involved in verbal or physical conflict. Some of the aides would show favoritism towards a resident, showering her

3

with special privileges. As material resources were scarce, this special treatment often resulted in the favored residents being attacked by their peers. A strategy for an attempt at control was to use the most feared resident at the top of the dominance hierarchy as an "enforcer," with the privilege of punishing others. Because the residents of these areas were being managed through isolation, intimidation, and punishment, little warmth and few attachments existed between them. Lack of interpersonal trust pervaded the environment.

As a special project, to strengthen and supplement an innovational behavioral program (Edmonson, Moxley & Nevil, 1980; Moxley, Nevil & Edmonson, 1980; Edmonson, Nevil & Moxley, 1980; Nevil & Edmonson, 1980) we planned the socialization game activities with a goal of shaping positive interaction between peers, and with a secondary goal of improving the interactions between the direct care staff and the residents. In part, this involved changing the negative valences that each person represented to the others into positive values. The methods we used via the games were basically those of desensitization, and of developing or strengthening social reinforcers such as attention and praise that could be used as contingencies for positive interpersonal behavior. Also, because of their years of depersonalization, games were used to make residents aware of their own attitudes and attributes in addition to those of others. Through trial of the games we invented, we discovered what was characteristic of the most successful, and it became continually easier to design additional activities.

Since our initial socialization game program, the therapeutic use of games has dramatically expanded. Our games have been used programmatically in vocational, school, and residential settings to focus on specific vocational or habilitation goals. We have also used games within individual and group counseling sessions to improve relationships among family members, peers, and caregivers. Numerous educators and practitioners have similarly expanded the application of the socialization game approach. *Game Play (1986)* was "the first state-of-the-art work" that focused on the psychological significance of using games with children and adolescents. The book featured sections on therapeutic socialization games for use with adolescents in group therapy; juveniles with delinquent behavior, and persons with mental retardation. More recently, Shapiro (1993) in *The Book of Psychotherapeutic Games* noted that hundreds of therapeutic games have been published since the mid 1980s. The popularity of the games appears to be due to many factors, including that they are easily learned, can be used by a wide range of professionals and paraprofessionals, and can be adapted to address most any need in any setting.

WHY USE THE GAMES?

We have found that socialization games are effective at holding the interest and attention of participants while they expand or try out a new behavioral repertoire. The laughter, the action, and the recognition that group members receive provide sufficient incentive to enable most individuals to learn skills ranging from basic group behaviors such as sitting and turn-taking to more complex group interactions such as interpersonal problem-solving and peer/team support.

The games are especially useful in promoting peer interdependence when the leader, after giving a demonstration, encourages the members to direct or to help one another in subsequent trials. Certain games are designed to require mutual assistance from the participants.

Socialization games are designed to enable all group members to feel like winners. In the games, players can be coached to better performance levels without their feeling they have failed at something. The warm and enthusiastic game leader, by focusing on the players' strengths and successes, helps to desensitize members to critical feedback and build self-confidence. There are no right or wrong responses, but only different or more effective ways to play. Playing the games can have a positive carryover effect on the interactions that group members have with others outside of the group. Generalization is, of course, more likely when other support people join the leader and the group members in the games. Through playing the games, the support people become more aware of socialization goals and their importance.

CHARACTERISTICS OF THE GAMES

As is more fully described in Section 5, the games focus on five socialization goal areas. The most basic set of games, interpersonal distance "Learning to be Close to Others," encourages group members to interact within close proximity. This socialization area is important in helping people with behavior problems learn to tolerate closeness to people whom they have not trusted in the past. In one of these games,

"Blow Round," participants sit closely together around a table in order to keep a ping pong ball from being blown off the table by others.

Another set of games has the goal of self-awareness or "Learning About Myself." In these games group members learn to identify their own feelings; learn how they feel about others' actions; and are encouraged to make independent choices and decisions. As an example, "I Feel Really Good About" requires participants to decide whether they feel good or bad in reaction to different situations.

A third set of games has the goal of social awareness or "Learning About Others." Several of these games, for example, require participants to learn about physical characteristics and personal preferences of others.

A fourth set of games focuses on prosocial behavior or "Learning to Get Along With Others" such as sharing, cooperation, helping, and mutual problem-solving. For example, in "I Have a Problem—How Can You Help?" participants are presented with a group member's problem and asked to suggest ways to help.

The fifth set of games, social competency or "Learning About Being A Part of My Community" focuses on how to engage in rule-governed and appropriate social behaviors, and to solve problems. Games in this category teach participants how to greet others, deal with anger, ask for help, and dress in a socially normative manner. "Something's Wrong with Those Clothes" teaches participants to discriminate problems with clothing. Participants then suggest ways of making the clothing look "OK". Some games in this category are used to develop problem-solving for members who have the necessary communicative and cognitive ability. Games such as "The Problem Box" involve members in considering problems that may occur in their environments—such as having something stolen, something lost, or something that needs repair. In some settings a member may have problems with money, loss of a job, or jealousy over a friend. Some of these games encourage members to think of alternative ways of resolving the problems.

The games lend themselves to many situations and purposes. After one has identified a socialization goal area, one can seek specific games in the scheme on pages 52–70. Games can be modified to fit particular persons or groups, or new games invented. While many of our games overlap goal areas, a primary goal should be evident in their design.

Group members may have special needs such as difficulty sitting still, paying attention, tolerating closeness of peers or controlling impulses. Some may have information processing problems which interfere with their ability to understand verbal directions. They may be hesitant to try something new, perhaps, because their failures have been emphasized more than their successes. Our socialization games, therefore, have been designed in terms of the following criteria:

Simplicity. Verbal explanations are minimized. Procedures are often communicated through modeling and imitation.

Novelty. Games frequently employ props, e.g., a timer, or stimulus cards, that can be used by group members, and which introduce an element of novelty.

Short Duration. Games move at a quick pace which tends to prevent satiation and sustain attention.

Participation. Many of the games promote active participation of all group members, throughout the session. For example, if two members are participating in a game in the middle of the group circle, other members have roles that may include counting, directing, voting or expressing an opinion about what is going on in the middle.

Turn-Taking. Each game includes a turn-taking procedure so that each member has an opportunity for individual participation during the session. This reduces competition over who is to have the next turn.

Success And Recognition. Social recognition is provided by the leader and other members for attempts to participate, for following the rules, completing steps of the activity, trying new strategies, and helping other members; thus, a participant has many opportunities to feel successful.

Cost. Games are designed to keep material cost and leader preparation time to a minimum. Many games require no materials. Most materials can be found among household or personal articles as with "Helping My Friend Find His/Her Stuff" or are easily made according to the directions in the game instructions.

Each game description includes the title, the goal area, the materials needed, the procedure, and the method for participant selection. The games are organized according to the group life phase (see Section 3; Tasks of the Group Leader) and the socialization goal area to which they pertain. Under the heading, Materials Needed, instructions are provided for any stimulus materials. Game procedures are simply stated and often include recommendations to guide the leader. With certain games there are additional suggestions for adapting or modifying the procedures. Since the games are relatively generic, leaders may want to make adaptations specific to member's ethnic, cultural and religious practices. For example, "I Know Something About You," "If I Were You" or "Signal If You Know" II may be easily modified to include examples of member practices (i.e., person was born in a different country, speaks a different language, wears different types of clothing, etc.).

The games can be used over and over again with different outcomes. Repetition seems to enhance effectiveness and interest value. As members become more familiar with the procedure, they can concentrate less on the rules and more on varying the outcome or their responses. Most games can be modified so the level of skill required to succeed can be gradually increased or adapted to fit the skill level of group members. Some of the games indicate advanced levels or second versions that require more skill. Most games can be easily adapted by the game leader to reduce or increase the level of difficulty. In the game "Find the Person" a simplified adaptation might require a participant to identify which of two persons has the object shown on the stimulus card. In an advanced version, members might be asked to classify or identify everyone in the group who has the object shown on the card. The leader may regard games as models or examples, and can experiment with modifications that address the socialization needs and interests of the group members.

RELEVANT POPULATIONS AND PROGRAMMATIC ENVIRONMENTS

The socialization games can be used with children, adolescents and adults in a variety of programs and environments. Although the games were initially designed for persons with moderate to severe mental retardation and challenging behaviors residing in a state-operated developmental center, they have been used successfully with persons of varying functional abilities and limitations in schools, vocational and psychiatric rehabilitation facilities, family homes, and a variety of group residential settings. The objectives and methods of the games are useful for improving personal and social adjustment, promoting inclusion and acceptance of differences and expanding recreational and leisure options.

Reference to the Game Assessment Scheme on pages (52–70) will suggest the relevance of particular games to certain groups. Furthermore, the classification system should help a program specialist identify some areas of habilitation need. After trial of the game designed for those areas, the group or game leader may think of modifications or new games that would be relevant.

SECTION 2

ORGANIZATIONAL AND
ENVIRONMENTAL REQUIREMENTS

A socialization game program involves the use of a group format. Thus, when developing a game program the group leader should be aware of factors that influence the behavior of a group. This section refers to important variables of group organization and physical environment that can effect group cohesiveness and behavior.

GROUP ORGANIZATION

Group organization is important to the outcome of the game program, as the group's organization will influence the ability of members to form interpersonal ties and to work cooperatively within the group.

Although there is limited research literature on the development of cohesion among group members with mental retardation or other disabilities, field trials of our games have shown an increase in friendly interactions and a decrease in unfriendly behavior consequent to the group experience (Han, 1980). Variables of group organization include: (1) the composition of the group; (2) the size of the group; (3) the basic rules for participation in the group; (4) the zones of participation in the group; (5) the length of a group session; and (6) the use of a time-limited group program. These are discussed below.

Composition

The question of *who* participates in a socialization game group may not be an option for a group leader whose clientele consists of persons grouped in a residential or vocational setting. In such an instance, the leader may have to work with an intact group consisting not only of individuals of all levels of functional abilities, but also perhaps of persons of different ages, and different levels of physical capabilities and

9

behavioral adjustment. Although such diversity makes group leadership difficult and decreases the habilitative impact of the game, this should not dissuade one from developing a game program. Many of the socialization games described in the final section of this book can be utilized with heterogeneous groups.

If a leader can select specific persons to become members of a socialization game group, we suggest that he/she consider the following criteria:

1. The sex of members is a significant variable of group composition. Many of the games can be utilized with same-sex or heterosexual groups. If a goal is to promote heterosexual interaction, then a group balanced with males and females should be developed. Same-sex groups might be considered when clients withdraw from members of the opposite sex; or need to develop peer interaction skills with members of their own gender.

2. The age of group members is another important variable. Although our experience has shown that the socialization games appeal to a broad age range of persons, a narrow age range may promote more group cohesion, because of members' similar developmental interests. A narrow age range may, thus, contribute to a group leader's goal of promoting peer relationships among group members.

3. The admixture of members of different functional abilities is an important variable. Our own experience has shown that a broad range of abilities creates challenges for the leader, because it is difficult to modify any single game so that it will sustain the interest and involvement of group members of widely discrepant abilities. In such an instance, the more able may be bored, or the least able may be virtually excluded from active involvement in group process. However, a group of persons of different functional levels within a narrow range can work with positive results. For several months, we conducted a group of women with moderate and severe mental retardation who resided in a state-operated developmental center. The women with moderate mental retardation were able to act as peer models and coaches for less able women. The latter gained much by observing the behavior of their peers and the more able were rewarded by their coaching role. A group leader may, therefore, want to seed the group with several persons who are functioning at a higher level than most group members. The greater the disparity in levels of functioning between group members, however; the more difficult or challenging it becomes for a group leader to provide success for all members.

4. Other variables that should be considered by the leader are the nature and extent of members' physical and behavioral challenges. Physical disability should not be cause for exclusion from the group, but the group leader must be sensitive to individuals' limitations and make adaptations in order to facilitate participation.

5. Behavior challenges are apt to be more problematic than physical disabilities to the leader who tries to achieve balanced group composition. The person who acts out aggressively should not be allowed to jeopardize the safety of others. On the other hand, because many of the games are designed to promote positive social behavior, one should not routinely and rigidly exclude people who may aggress, as they need opportunities to acquire more adaptive social skills. When persons with serious behavior problems are included, the leader must set limits, and must find ways of holding their interest to promote a progressive decline in disruptive behavior.

6. Another variable effecting group organization is the participation in the group by support staff. When we lead a group, we encourage participation by support persons, since many group members have developed positive relationships with these staff. This only reinforces the importance of the group, and also encourages the concept of having fun while learning valuable social skills.

To summarize, differences in group composition can have a profound effect on the behavior and attitude of individual members, and leaders should be aware of the characteristics of members that differentially influence the functioning of groups. If leaders have the option of selecting members they should plan in terms of the following variables: (1) gender; (2) age; (3) level of functioning capabilities; (4) physical capabilities; (5) behavior/emotional difficulties; and (6) the possible inclusion of support persons. If the leader does not have control over these variables then he or she will need to consider how the characteristics of group members may effect group process and plan accordingly.

Size

Group size should vary according to whether one or two group leaders are involved, and according to the challenges and related needs for support presented by individual group members. We have found the decision matrix presented in Figure 1 to be useful in planning the size of the group.

Level of Challenges/Need for Supports

		Low	*High*
	1	4–6	3–4
Number of Leaders			
	2	8–10	6–8

Figure 1. Decision matrix for planning size of game group.

The cells indicate the number of members that we recommend in relation to the number of leaders and the incidence of challenges presented by the group. When one leader is working with a group with low support needs, a range of from four to six members is suggested, while a range of from three to four members is suggested for a group with a higher need for support. The size of the group and the decision whether to have two leaders should be influenced by the functional abilities of group members and the nature of any physical and behavioral challenges presented by group members. Two leaders are better able to accommodate a higher incidence of challenges, but must carefully assess the impact on other group members. Given two leaders and a low support need, an ideal size is from eight to ten members.

Basic Rules for Participation

Another organizational variable consists of the basic rules for group participation. These rules should be identified and discussed with the group at the beginning of the socialization game program. Rules might include: (1) Group members will take turns talking (2) Group members will treat each other with respect (i.e., listening, keeping hands to ones self, using friendly words), (3) Group members will cooperate and help each other. Leaders may need to assist the members with understanding the reasons for the rules by giving examples of both appropriate and inappropriate behaviors in a game-like scenario. For example, the leader(s) can take turns demonstrating members talking at the same time, getting in and out of seats, making noise while others are taking turns, and other disruptive behaviors. Members can then choose their own rules based on their respective ratings of the behaviors. Some members may need occasional reminders and/or redirection by the leader to maintain appropriate group behavior. In some cases, additional intervention by the leader may be necessary to defuse or support a member's behavior. The goal is to preserve the group and even brief exclusion of a member should be a last resort.

Zones of Participation

We conceive of two zones of participation as constituting another aspect of the organization of a group. The first zone or the "core group" are the members, seated in a circle, who are involved in face-to-face interaction in the group. The second zone, the "outfield," consists of those who sit or stand on the fringe or edge of the group and watch the activity of the core members. We have observed that some persons, because of negativism or aversion to physical proximity, resist becoming involved in the core group. We encourage such persons to sit nearby and watch. From time to time the leaders are able to get the individuals to respond to a question or participate, even if briefly, with the core group. This participation, vicarious or direct, by reluctant persons should be encouraged as it can lead to learning and to eventual core group participation.

Length of A Group Session

Sessions should be structured to take into account members' attention spans. The length of a session is a critical factor in maintaining positive interaction within the group. Once group members become bored or otherwise inattentive, positive interaction decreases and some members may withdraw from the group or begin to be disruptive. During the group pilot program, it appeared that an optimal session ranged from 30 to 45 minutes. This time span was sufficient for "getting ready," playing a game, and "cooling down." For groups with members who have developed group prerequisite skills (i.e., sitting, attending, waiting), sessions have been effectively expanded to 50–90 minutes.

Time-Limited Programming

This final organizational variable involves planning for the life span of the group. Time-limited groups are an option for group leaders such as psychologists, counselors, social workers, teachers, or activity therapists who must provide group programs for a large number of persons for a limited period of time. Short-term game groups might range from

10 to 12 sessions and have a specific focus/goal. Some of the areas of focus that we have addressed have included:

1. "Learning About Each Other" or a series of group sessions designed to help new roommates become acquainted.

2. "Getting Along" or a series of group sessions designed to help members learn conflict resolution and interpersonal problem-solving.

3. "Being a Responsible Worker/Making It at My Job" or a series of group sessions designed to help workers learn to deal with work adjustment issues in a new job setting.

4. "Learning About My Feelings and Behavior" or a series of sessions to help promote insight and self awareness.

5. "Keeping Myself Safe" or a series of sessions designed to promote self-awareness related to personal safety issues.

6. "Being A Responsible Friend" ("Special Friendships") or a series of sessions to help deal with the responsible issues of friendships/relationships.

7. "I love you!" or a series of group sessions to help couples improve communication.

Examples of group programs focusing on conflict resolution and work adjustment will be described in more detail in section #4.

GROUP ENVIRONMENT

The physical environment is influential in maintaining the organization of the game group. Variables that should be considered by the group leader include: (1) characteristics of the room; (2) environmental distractions; (3) type of furniture and its arrangements; (4) useful "props;" and (5) scheduling group time.

Characteristics of the Physical Space

The room should be large enough to accommodate the group sitting in a circle formation. For some games additional space may be needed. Ideally, the space utilized for socialization games should not be overly large. If a large room must be utilized, the game area boundaries should be clearly denoted with tables or screens or chairs.

The most important guideline is that the same room or meeting areas be used each time. The familiar setting helps members remember the procedural rules and pleasurable experiences and creates within members an expectation of fun that optimizes their attentiveness and effort.

Controlling Environmental Distractors

A group leader wants members to focus their attention on what is happening within the core group. Factors that divert attention from group involvement include large windows; noise from telephones, television, radios, or tape or CD players; nonparticipating persons entering and leaving the area; and extremes in room temperature. Distractors can often be prevented or minimized. In certain environments, however, the group leader may have to manage with limited control over distractions. For example, in sheltered workshops it may not be possible or practical to move a group due to transportation issues, time constraint, lack of space, or member resistance. We have been surprised at our member's continuing interest and ability to focus on the games despite multiple distractions. The group leader's efforts to manage the environment should help to maintain good group interaction.

Type of Furniture and its Arrangement

Because the games are intended to increase physical and social contact between members, the furniture that is used is important. Couches and sofas encourage members to sit next to one another, but there should be comfortable (and movable) chairs for those who avoid physical proximity. Group participants might sit on the floor on overstuffed pillows, but members with physical challenges or poor motor control may be limited by this arrangement. The important consideration is to use furniture that will be comfortable for the duration of the group session.

An effective arrangement of furniture is an open-ended circle. This allows props, (e.g., a small table or chair) to be moved in and out of the group with minimal disruption of group activity, while allowing members to conveniently move in and out of the center of the circle as required by certain games.

Use of Props

Many of the socialization games require props. These may be extra chairs, a table, containers, timers or index cards. In order to avoid disruption of the group, these props should be set up or moved to the periphery of the group before beginning the game session.

Scheduling Group Time

In scheduling group games, leaders should choose a day and time that does not conflict with meals and responsibilities, e.g., school, chores, work, field trips. Our experience has shown that scheduling groups just prior to mealtimes or too late in the evenings interferes with group process and outcome. Once a time is selected, the leader should attempt to maintain this as the regular group time. This will give members some predictability. Members will then become secure and confident that their group will be held at a set day and time. This consistency allows group members to anticipate and prepare for their participation in the group process.

SECTION 3

GROUP LEADERSHIP

The role of the group leader is a challenging and often demanding job, but is certainly not limited to those with extensive training or expertise. Leadership and effective group management skills develop from the experience one gains by actually conducting groups. It is important, then, to "take the plunge" and start working with a group on the assumption that you, as the leader, will grow with the group members. The focus of this section is on group leadership: leadership characteristics, leadership goals and general techniques, and the tasks of the group leader, including many specific techniques for promoting group involvement and cohesion.

GENERAL CHARACTERISTICS OF A GROUP LEADER

The leader should be aware of certain leadership characteristics or behaviors that appear to be necessary for effective group management. These are: (1) demonstrating enthusiasm, (2) conveying warmth, (3) communicating effectively, and (4) promoting trust.

Demonstrating Enthusiasm. The group leader is a powerful role model for group members. Members will not only model or imitate what the leader explains and demonstrates, but will also model the mood he or she conveys. It is, thus, essential for the leader to express enthusiasm and interest in the group activities. If not, the members may lose or never develop interest. The leader creates the mood and sets the tone for group activities. A principle goal is to be as enthusiastic about the activities as you expect your members to be.

It is often helpful to emphasize and even exaggerate your interest both verbally, and nonverbally with gestures. We have had group members who initially thought that the games were childish or foolish, but who then decided the games were fun in reaction to our enthusiasm.

Warmth. The leader must convey warmth, acceptance and recognition. Warmth and concern are conveyed through verbal statements, body

17

language, facial expression, and physical gestures. Warmth is expressed in many ways, but includes such gestures as; greeting, and if necessary, shaking hands with each member, praising individuals and the group as a whole for their participation, and showing special consideration for members' problems or concerns. While the group game session is not group therapy designed to focus on members' personal problems, a sensitive and warm leader should give special attention to members with concerns, and encourage others in the group to provide support. We have found that if a member is upset before a group session, but made to feel accepted and needed by the group and leader, he/she will often have a change of mood and be able to put aside the upsetting situation. Thus, the group session can provide a comfortable atmosphere and promote positive feelings toward self and others.

Communication. Effective communication is essential in establishing and maintaining groups that work. The leader must be highly conscious of his/her verbal and nonverbal messages and of the receptive and expressive abilities of group members. Through initial questions and trial activities, members' levels of understanding can be assessed.

When introducing the games, the leader can use a combination of verbal instructions and physical modeling, to be repeated as necessary. For members who appear unable to follow lengthy or complex verbal directions, game procedures may have to be broken down into simple steps, and each step rehearsed or "walked through" before proceeding on to the next. Adaptation of instructions and demonstration are important techniques to facilitate or promote learning.

Trust. The group leader can be an effective facilitator of positive interaction only if he/she has earned the members' trust. Trust can be promoted when groups are conducted regularly on a certain day at a set time. Group members may feel more secure if they can expect groups to occur on a set schedule. It is also important that the leader consistently enforces the rules. Rules for acceptable conduct were made for the benefit of the group and need to be followed if the leader is to be trusted and effective.

As a model, the leader can make mistakes intentionally to show members that "It is OK to make a mistake." This model of human fallibility lessens members' concerns about mistakes and failure, thereby reducing performance pressure. Members can also be asked to inform the leader if he/she makes a mistake which equalizes the balance of power and enhances mutual trust.

LEADERSHIP GOALS AND GENERAL TECHNIQUES

The group leader's primary role is to help members develop positive interactions with one another. When members interact positively with one another in the group without being prompted to do so by the leader, the likelihood is increased that such behaviors will transfer to situations outside of the group. Han's data (1980) supports the effectiveness of the group game approach as she found that significantly more friendly interactions occurred immediately following the group games than after a variety of other structured group activities.

With some newly organized groups, a first goal of the leader will be to teach members to listen and to sit in a group formation. In the beginning phase of group involvement, the leader must be highly didactic, reinforcing, and involved in order to establish the basic rules for participation. As the members learn to play the games and follow the rules, the leader increases the members' responsibility by assuming a less directive posture. Gradually, the leader works toward the group members' helping one another.

To increase individual responsibility and enhance the attraction of the group, the leader must determine what behaviors to reinforce and how to reinforce them. Two major categories of behavior that should be reinforced are positive social interaction and self-directed behavior. Positive social interaction includes cooperative behavior such as sitting quietly and waiting for a turn, following the group rules, and members helping one another or praising one another for their efforts. The leader can promote positive interaction by offering members opportunities to help him or her and to help other members. Through shaping techniques, a members' social repertoire can be expanded from simple social interactions to a self-directed level. At this level, members no longer wait for requests from the leader, but, for example, sit quietly and follow their rules. They may begin to offer assistance spontaneously and initiate other positive interactions.

Reinforcement consists of verbal and nonverbal recognition and praise. Recognition and praise of group members' efforts should consistently come from the leader, but can be even more effective when coming from the group. The leader teaches members to "recognize" and reinforce one another. We often demonstrate praise by hand clapping or gesturing "thumbs up" for members' performance. Group members first follow the leader's cue and eventually discriminate appropriate reinforcement times without relying on the leader. Verbal praise follows a similar course, as initially, group members imitate the leader and then spontaneously praise others. Teaching members to look for and publicly recognize the efforts of others promotes growth from an egocentric perspective to a higher level of social awareness. Some of our most egocentric members have learned to look beyond themselves and exhibit excitement over the successes of others. We have seen one such member pat another on the back and exclaim, "I'm so proud of you."

Mutually helpful and self-directed behavior should be goals of the group leader. It will require conscious effort to foster the members' reliance on peers and on self rather than on the leader. One technique is to redirect members who need assistance to peers, rather than responding to these needs. Members can also be encouraged to solve their own problems by using graduated prompting. With this technique, rather than solving a problem, the leader prompts an answer or suitable response with a series of questions.

To promote goals of peer helpfulness and self-directed behavior, the leader should allow members to direct themselves as much as they can and will. When the leader must assist, the method of intervention is important. His or her attempts should be to guide via prompting, insofar as feasible, rather than by a direct demonstration or a full explanation. If a member cannot recall what it is that he or she is supposed to be doing, or has difficulty with the activity, the leader can prompt the procedural steps. For example, if Linda has not been able to locate the group member with a design that matches her own for the "Match Game," the leader might first ask Linda and then the group, "Did you/she look at everyone's design?" The leader prompts the group to respond with "No" or a headshake. The leader could then ask another member to help Linda walk around the group and as the pair stops at each member, the leader could guide with questions; e.g., "Did you look at Mary's?" "Does yours look like Mary's?" and so on. The leader could encourage the peer helper and others to assist with additional questions as necessary. In this way, the leader encourages both problem-solving and peer assistance.

Group members are also prompted to give assistance to members with situations that are unrelated to specific game activities. For example, if a member has a physical disability that limits his/her involvement or mobility, others are encouraged to assist, but not to *do* the activity for that member. Even individuals with severely limiting conditions can assist others in some way. It is the responsibility of the group leader to encourage the contributions and assistance of each member based on his/her individual ability. Every member should discover that he/she can be a valuable contributor to the group.

Group leaders should encourage members to generate their own ideas. For instance, during the "Greeting Game," members are encouraged to come up with their own examples of "weird" and "OK" behaviors. We have found that members functioning in the low-moderate to severe range of mental retardation are often able to come up with their own ideas with prompting. If a member can give an example of "weird" or "OK" behaviors, he or she is developing discrimination abilities.

TASKS OF THE GROUP LEADER

Planning for Phases of Group Life

Groups begin; grow with respect to planned goals; and then end. To accommodate these three identifiable phases of group life, games have been designed to address the needs specific to each phase, which we refer to as the Warm-Up Phase, the Game Phase and the Closing Phase.

Warm-Up Phase

With beginning groups made up of members who lack basic group skills, the emphasis is on getting members interested and enthused about the group experience and teaching basic group skills. The leader focuses on the fun value of the game while teaching members to sit in a group, maintain attention, follow directions, respect rules, and take turns. Games designed for the Warm-Up Phase are action-oriented and require imitative responses rather than more advanced cognitive skills.

The leader gauges the readiness of group members to move on to the Game Phase by observing their interest level and group-skill level. Depending upon the duration of the group and the needs of group members, the leader decides when the group is able to handle games addressing specific socialization goal areas. Some groups, meeting for a short duration, with members who have great difficulty coping with the demands of the group process, may remain in the Warm-Up Phase until the end of the group program. Group leaders are encouraged to try games in the interpersonal distance goal area as these games tend to promote a fairly high degree of member involvement. Also, some warm-up games address the area of learning about others. These games are especially useful for beginning groups as they encourage members to learn about others in the group. The important point is that members' behavior will communicate to the leader whether the phase or particular game is appropriate.

Game Phase

The majority of the games are designed to improve skills in the five general socialization areas detailed in Section 2. Some games place more cognitive demand on members and require the ability to remain seated and wait for a turn because only one or two can play at a time.

Most groups spend the bulk of their sessions in the Game Phase working on goals prioritized by the leader to meet the needs of the group members. As games within each socialization area represent a range of difficulty levels, a leader may want to concentrate on a particular goal area before moving on to another. For example, a leader may focus on decreasing interpersonal distance through relevant games before moving on to games promoting social awareness or social competency.

Leaders should not, however, feel limited to a single socialization area and may instead want to rotate games among the socialization areas. Again, the critical task for the leader is to select games that meet the needs and skill levels of group members.

Closing Phase

The Closing Phase of group life is designed to provide a positive group ending to the group experience so that members will feel less wary about their involvement in future groups. All too often, groups simply stop with an announcement at the final session; or, even worse, members discover, after the fact, that their group has been discontinued. Members are then left with no understanding as to the reason for the ending and may be left with a multitude of negative feelings such as anger, sadness, rejection or personal inadequacy. We feel that a sensitive leader *must* consider the feelings of members about their group and in so doing prepare members for the conclusion of the experience. Whether the group is time-limited or ongoing, the end is inevitable. It is recommended that closing procedures be planned and implemented prior to the final session to permit leaders and members some time to work through their feelings and adjust to the ending of the group.

The games that are appropriate for the closing phase are designed to sensitize group members to the approaching ending of the game program. Closing games provide participants with opportunities to express their feelings and attitudes about the end of the group experience. Some games help members plan for activities after the group program is completed. Although members may not become involved in such activities, these games communicate the leader's interest in members continuing to interact with one another even though the game program has ended.

We recommend that the leader arrange the time frame so that the group begins the closing process three sessions prior to the final session. For groups with members who have poor communication skills, the leader can adapt the process by omitting the first session. The recommended session outline follows:

Session I. Prior to playing the game, members are involved in a discussion about their thoughts and feelings related to the group. The leader may facilitate discussion with structured questions such as:

- What is your favorite game?
- What do you like best about our group?
- Are there any things you don't like about the group?
- How would you improve or make the group better?

Each member is given the opportunity to respond to questions about the group. The leader then announces that group will meet two more times, and provides members with an explanation for the ending of the group. If the group was time-limited the leader may remind the members weekly "This is our 5th/6th/7th group, we will meet 10/9/8 more times." Then, closing becomes the final part of the countdown. For open-ended groups however, the leader needs to explain to members the reason for the group coming to a close. It may be that the leader is giving others an opportunity to participate in a group or that the leader is changing roles or jobs. Whatever the reason, members should be informed and given the opportunity to react. Members also need to know the leader's feelings about the group and the impending ending. The session then becomes an exchange of feelings and thoughts between leaders and members.

Session II. This part of the closing process consists of a ritual, or the playing of games designed to facilitate movement towards closure. The games provide a structured format for expression of feelings and thoughts about the group. The leader reminds members that the following session will be the last group session.

Session III. The final session can include both a group ritual and group product. Members could be asked to select a piece of construction paper and pen/marker. Each member then makes a card for another group member selected by drawing a name or picture. The session is concluded with the leader presenting his/her card to the group. If possible, leaders might also take pictures of the group for each member to keep as a concrete reminder of the group experience.

If realistic, leaders may also tell members that even though the group will no longer be meeting, the leaders will try to maintain contact from time to time. It is important that a leader attempt to minimize members' feelings of rejection by helping them focus on positive outcomes from the group experience (e.g., friends made, favorite games or activities, special memories).

Planning the Group Session

Each group session may be divided into three parts: (1) "Getting Ready," (2) "Game Time," and (3) "Summing Up." For a 30–45 minute game session we suggest 5 minutes for Part 1, 20–30 minutes for Part 2 and 5–10 minutes for Part 3. The duration of phases should be determined by the number of players, their interests, and their needs.

"Getting Ready" permits leaders to promote group identity by using some of the suggested techniques to prepare members for the game. The leader may want to remind members of the group rules and procedures that will be used during the game session. For example, a leader might hold up a prop and elicit from members the rules regarding it's use. Also, group member responsibilities such as being a peer helper or in charge of rearranging the furniture could be delegated. To assist members with focusing, it is often helpful to review or discuss the previous session's activities.

Once the attention of members has been established through "Getting Ready," the leader shifts into "Game Time." The game is introduced through a modeling demonstration and all members have opportunities to play as suggested in sections titled "Phases of Group Life" and "Introduction of the Games."

"Summing Up" is a time in which to review the session and reinforce members for their participation. The review could include a brief description of the game, individual member contributions, specific strategies discussed, or other closing thoughts. Members are also rewarded by special recognition for their participation. The leader tells group members that they have done a great job and worked well together as a group and reminds them of their next group meeting time.

A leader may also want to involve all members in an activity to provide closure to the game session. One technique is the group "vote." The leader asks, "Everyone who likes playing (*name of game*), signal or raise your hand." Group members can assist by counting the votes. The "vote" method encourages members to state a preference and recognize differences in preferences. When the activity is repeated, the leader should remind members, "We are playing (*name of game*) again because the group chose to play it." Thus, the group members are shown that their preferences or choices within the group are meaningful and important.

Preparing Members for Game Session

While groups may be conducted "at a moment's notice," there are many advantages to scheduling them at regular times. Groups scheduled to occur on a specific day at a certain time promote an awareness of time. When members expect the session as a regularly occurring event, they can anticipate and prepare for it, thus becoming more self-directed and ready for responsible participation.

The program staff or support persons can prepare members by reminding them of the day and time of their session at intervals during the week if possible and several minutes before the group is scheduled to begin. As an example, a support person can say, "Your group meets Tuesdays at 5:30," or "Your group will meet in 10 minutes." To remind members ahead of time rather than to request their participation at the time of the sessions, allows them to assume the responsibility for being ready.

Getting People to the Group

For individuals who appear disinterested and for those who actively refuse to participate in the group, a follow-up prompting procedure is often effective. The following 3-step procedure must be approached positively:

1. The leader or a support person says, "We would like you to come to the group."
2. The individual is reminded that he/she is important to the group. For example, "You do (could do) such a good job. We really need you to help us in the group." The message is that the member has alot to offer and is valued by the other group members.
3. If the individual refuses, he/she is told, "When you are ready to come to the group or play the games, please let me know."

Some members respond well to being given a special job or an assisting role as an incentive for coming to the group. This procedure should be used only initially to permit that person to have some successful experiences. The assisting role can then be rotated to others. It is the leader's responsibility to make the group rewarding enough to maintain the members' interest. We have found that most members will continue to attend once they have participated in a fun session.

It is important that the group begin on time with or without all members. While the member who initially refuses to attend may join at any time, he/she must see that the group will not wait. Individuals usually do not like to miss out on the fun that they see others having in the group.

Introduction of Games

The leader introduces a game by demonstration. We have developed a four-step modeling strategy for introducing group games:

1. The leader introduces the game by announcing its name and simple concrete instructions for playing. If materials are involved, the leader may want to acquaint the members with them using a questioning procedure. For example, if a blindfold is used, the leader can ask group members if they can identify the object and then encourage a member to demonstrate its use.
2. The leader "walks through" the game procedure.
3. The leader selects a member and uses prompting to begin the game.
4. Group members play the game with the leader providing direct guidance and prompting.

Once a game has been played by the group, it can usually be reintroduced by presenting the materials and basic directions. Through questioning, the leader can determine the extent of members' recall and can adapt the procedures accordingly. With repetition, the members learn the games and can then provide assistance as peer facilitators.

Maintaining Formation of the Group

Many strategies are used by the leader to maintain the attention and interest of the group members. Close circular arrangement of the chairs or cushions promotes proximity of the members and facilitates attention to one another. The activities are designed to promote active involvement of group members so that they will want to remain in the group. Most important, however, are the skills and techniques of the group leader in maintaining group cohesion.

The effective group leader has the dual role of "planner" and "scanner." As a "planner," the leader must organize and direct the activities so as to permit the active involvement of all members. In addition, the leader must be a "scanner" throughout the group sessions for situations that threaten to disrupt the group process, and be prepared to follow through with planned intervention techniques. The leader can maximize group cohesion and prevent disruptions by using the following techniques:

Turn Taking. Explain to members that they will have a turn to participate. One method of turn taking is called "BLIND SELECTION." Members' names or pictures are drawn, one at a time, to determine who has the next turn. This method gives everyone an equal chance of being selected. It eliminates favoritism and promotes the attention of group members through anticipation of being next.

Another turn-taking procedure is the "LEADER SELECTION" method during which the leader chooses members. The advantage of this selection method lies in the flexibility afforded to the leader. The leader may simply rotate participation by seating order or choose members based on circumstances. For example, members who are distracted or distracting others may be selected and, thus, redirected to the activity when necessary.

Rotating Attention. Attention focused too long on a single member can often result in losing the attention of the rest of the group. The leader can maintain the attention of all group members by switching his/her focus from member to member, or by rotating attention around the group. It is important that the flow of reciprocal interactions from leader to member to leader to another member, be maintained to keep all members interested and involved throughout the session.

Paradoxical Prompting. To increase members' attending behavior and facilitate active participatory learning, we often present a verbal paradox or false statement to group members. A paradoxical statement may be a misstatement of group rules or game procedures such as, "Let's all talk at the same time?" or "Let's just sleep instead of playing a game." The purpose of such statements is to encourage members' active listening and correction of the statement rather than blind acceptance of leader's remarks. As members learn to respond discriminatively to leader's statements, the leader is also able to gauge the member's comprehension of game rules and procedures.

Shaping members' discrimination of false statements requires that the leader encourage members to listen carefully to repetition of the statements and actively guide them through questioning to recognize the inaccuracy. Initially, our members required considerable prompting to challenge leader statements. With practice and improved listening skills, however, members learned to discriminate the false statements with a resounding *"No"* followed by a corrected statement.

Maintaining Focus On Activity. Group members may want to talk about personal needs or concerns for which the group session is not the appropriate time or place. The effective leader uses redirection techniques. Consequently, when Linda begins to talk about the money she was given, the leader can respond by first acknowledging the issue or concern and then refocusing Linda. For example, "Linda, let's talk about that after the group."

Physical Support. Physical support consists of contact such as patting an arm or shoulder, giving a "high five," or special handshake as encouragement or reinforcement for participating in the group. Through physical support, the group leader can communicate acceptance, support, or praise for a job well done. The leader using physical support is also a social model demonstrating acceptable touching to group members.

Recognition of Cooperative Behavior. The leader can promote group process by reinforcing the group for working together. It is important to give verbal recognition and support to members for cooperative behavior with such statements as "Everyone works together as a team in this group", or "You are all doing a great job together," or "See how well we help each other." Group members should be encouraged to assist each other on an individual basis and to provide group support by clapping or cheering for others' efforts. The message is that the group is a supportive team and that each member contributes to the group's activity.

Promoting Group Identity. A major task for the leader is to promote "we" feelings among group members or a sense of group togetherness. Members are encouraged to see themselves and the other members as forming a distinct group that is identifiable from other groups in terms of purpose and expectations. Beyond identifying one's membership in a given group, members need to feel positive about their roles if the group experience is to be influential. There is much evidence to show that the more attractive a group is to it's members, the greater the positive influence members and leaders will have on one another.

Groups acquire an identity and positive valence, or attractiveness through the efforts of the leader. Most basically, the leader promotes the identity of the group by designating a particular theme and structured routine (set time, place and membership composition). Members then learn that they and some of their peers are part of a regularly occurring special event different from other daily group activities.

The unique identity of the group primarily comes from the nature of the activities. Members need to know why they are coming to the group and what is expected of them as members. Giving the group a name such as "Friendship Group" or "Responsible Worker Group" enhances group identity by giving members a common label reflecting the purpose of the group. We often begin and conclude our groups with a ritual in which the leader asks all members of the "Game Group" to respond to questions such as: "Who remembers the name of our group?" and "When do we meet?" and "What are we here to talk about?" As members learn to verbalize (or sign) together the name, topic and day their group meets, they tend to feel a greater sense of belonging and identification with each other as members of the same group. Concrete symbols such as game prop box or group member folders may also serve to promote group identity as they present unique materials specific to the group focus.

Group members express their feelings about the group basically through their willingness to participate in group activities. Other indicators of members' perception of group identity are member's questions and comments about the group between sessions. Some of our groups have gathered together before each session without prompting and talked among themselves and to others about their group activities. In addition, members of some of the groups have continued to ask support staff even years later if they could be in another group.

Reinforcement. For group members needing considerable support to cope with the group structure, it may be helpful to use planned reinforcement. For example, members who have difficulty entering the group, sitting, or staying within the group areas could be given contingent reinforcers such as praise, tokens or snacks. In the beginning, it's important to reinforce on a more frequent basis. Gradually the reinforcers are decreased or faded as members learn to cope with the group structure and rules.

Minimizing Distractors. Members talking among themselves can be very disruptive to the group process. We have used several methods for quieting disruptive group members. Members of one of our groups who had a hard time controlling their talking were taught to take turns cueing others in the group. In time, group members can assume the responsibility of monitoring and controlling the noise level.

The leader must also be able to maintain or regain the attention of the group members who are obviously distracted or upset. The leader must be an active "scanner" to watch for members who seem frustrated. Quick intervention using redirection techniques is often effective at defusing the upset member. Often a positive comment or question about the individual's performance is sufficient. A proactive method is to assign the member a specific task. One very disruptive individual who threatened and assaulted others outside of the group responded positively when given the role of holding the game materials.

If group members are involved as helpers throughout the session, behavior management problems are reduced. When members are busy, they are more interested and less apt to feel frustrated. Not all members will respond at all times to redirection. If a member is nonviolent, but disrupting the group, we suggest a four-step prompting procedure. First, the individual is told, "We can't hear what Jim is saying. Can you please help us out by being quiet?," and given an opportunity to gain control of his/her behavior. If the behavior persists, the member is asked, "Do you need some time away from the group?" If the behavior continues, then the individual is reminded of the contingency, "If you cannot be quiet, and respect others, you will have to leave the group." Finally, if the above steps are unsuccessful, the individual is told, "You must leave the group, but you may come back when you are ready." Continuing disruptive behavior results in an escort away from the group. It is important to remind the member that when he or she is ready he/she can rejoin the group. This is not a punishment, but an opportunity to get behavior under control. For violent behavior, an immediate intervention is necessary to protect other group members. The guiding principle for ruling on disruptive behavior is: How much can the group tolerate and still remain safe and focused on the task?

Attention of group members may also wane if an activity is perceived too complicated, boring or uninteresting. The leader views the group's mood and behavior as a barometer of the interest value of a specific game. When signs of group boredom or satiation occur, such as increased fidgeting and talking, the leader needs to assess the situation and be prepared to modify or change the activity. Group members may provide information in response to questions from the leader that will assist him/her in making successful adaptations.

Co-Leadership

A helpful strategy is to enlist the assistance of a co-leader. Two co-leaders can more effectively demonstrate game procedures and provide role-modeling of social interactions. The additional energy generated by a co-leader also enhances the potential involvement and enthusiasm of group members as well as allowing leaders to rotate responsibilities. Leader expertise and capabilities can be further expanded by teaming leaders from different disciplines or areas of specialization. For example, communication specialists could team with other professionals to assist group members with special communication needs. Two leaders, working as a team, are especially helpful with group members who exhibit challenging behaviors.

While co-leaders will necessarily overlap in terms of their responsibilities, direction of the games and supporting behavior represent two different roles. One co-leader can be primarily responsible for directing the game while the other can assume primary responsibility for group maintenance and behavior support techniques as was previously mentioned. The leaders maintain an unobtrusive communication dialogue mostly on a nonverbal basis so that each can supplement and assist the other. It is important that the leaders are consistent with one another in their communication with group members.

The co-leader approach is especially important for individuals with challenging behavior as some require almost one-to-one support to adapt to the group expectations. As an example, in one of our groups a new member initially spent most of her time wandering around trying to grab things from other members. It required the skillful efforts of one leader to shape her sitting behavior and to prompt her participation while the co-leader kept the game going with the other members. Once members learn to follow group rules, it is possible to fade one co-leader and continue the group with a single leader.

Not all group leaders, of course, have the option of a co-leader. If one is to work alone with individuals who display challenging behavior, a careful assessment of the characteristics of the members and the limitations of a single group leader is in order as indicated in Section 2. Strategies include limiting the size of the group and selecting adaptive peers as models and helpers.

This section on group leadership was developed to prepare support staff to become more effective group leaders by orienting them to their roles and providing helpful suggestions and strategies for maximizing group cohesion and member growth. Prospective leaders should view the facilitation strategies as procedures which have been found to be useful with some groups, but which should be adapted to meet the needs of particular group members. Leaders are urged to use these techniques as the basis for the development of their own strategies.

Applications

Since the initial printing of "Socialization Games," we have significantly expanded the focus and range of applications of the games. Although we have not formally conducted research on the effectiveness of the games, we have received numerous reports related to their usefulness and appeal from persons providing services in the areas of mental retardation and developmental disabilities, mental health, neurological rehabilitation and health care. Some of the settings/situations in which we have found the games to be particularly useful have included supported living and supported employment. As many adults with mental retardation and/or other disabilities have entered these types of situations, the need and demand for improved social behavior has been critical to their success. Adjustment has been even more difficult for those individuals coming from institutional, restrictive or impoverished environments.

We have found games to be particularly helpful with those individuals challenged by multiple or sensitive adjustment issues. Since games are fun and impersonal, they reduce the potential threat of confronting the issues. Group members tend to feel more comfortable problem-solving and talking about difficulties. For example, games have been used to facilitate improved worker or employee attitudes and behavior, such as acceptance of supervision and conflict resolution with peers. We will describe group socialization programs in the next section involving the use of games to increase participant's awareness and skills in the areas of adjustment issues related to competitive employment and shared living.

SECTION 4

DESIGNING SOCIALIZATION GAMES
AND GROUP PROGRAMS

While our games can provide you with enough material for hours of socialization, half of the fun comes with designing your own games and group programs. This section provides guidelines, strategies and group program outlines to assist the beginning group leader.

We have recently been involved with developing and implementing group programs for individuals experiencing difficulties in their work or home environments. For these groups, efforts were made to individualize the games to focus on identified issues and concerns. We offer three of these socialization group programs as examples. Based on your group members and leaders availability, the structured activities and number of sessions may be reduced or expanded as needed. Sessions also may be repeated periodically for review purposes or if new issues arise. We encourage you to individualize and create games and programs that focus on or address your own special needs and interests.

DESIGNING THE GAMES

When designing games, we suggest the following questions and considerations to guide you through the process. As you become more experienced and comfortable with developing games for your group members, the process will become easier and less deliberate.

1. Assess your groups' needs and strengths related to motor, sensory, and cognitive functioning. Are members able to move easily or are physical movements limited? Do members have visual or auditory difficulties that would necessitate specialized procedures? Are members cognitively capable of problem-solving or are methods such as matching and motor imitation more appropriate?

2. Assess your groups' needs or issues and identify a goal area such as prosocial behavior ("learning to get along with others"). What are

34

you trying to teach or help the members learn? What are the basic discriminations that will facilitate learning?

3. Assess your groups special interests (i.e., hobbies, sports, TV programs, music, etc.). How can these interest areas be used within the game format to address the goal area?

4. Determine roles for leaders and members. Can group members maintain their attention while individuals take turns or do group members need more frequent opportunities to participate?

5. Identify materials that could be easily obtained to provide novelty and cues/prompts for participation. What creative approaches can you use to make the activity fun and interesting?

6. Describe the step-by-step procedures for playing the game. How will the game be introduced? How will members participate (one at a time; two at a time; together as a group)? How will the materials be used? What will be the members' objective? How will the leader participate (i.e., hand out materials; actively prompt member responses; facilitate discussion)? Based on the identified issues and discriminations to be taught, what situations or scenarios could be used?

We recently were asked to design a game for a group of employees in a sheltered workshop. Using the above process questions and considerations, we determined that based on their motor, sensory and cognitive functional abilities, ideal games would involve motor imitation and concrete concepts and directions. Since group member interactions were limited, the Socialization Goal was to increase prosocial behavior. Due to the interest of members in Special Olympics and the concurrent preparation for the summer games, we decided to use the sports theme. We then developed a game procedure by first identifying a list of various team sports including rowing, tennis, basketball, volleyball, etc. We next devised a turn-taking procedure involving the selection of small groups of members who would demonstrate a particular team sport. Other members would be asked to guess the sport. These procedures permitted a high level of involvement and participation with virtually no material cost.

We have found that games simply must be played or tried out in order to determine if they work or not with a specific group. Sometimes group members will come up with game modifications, or their own versions, after they are familiar with the game concept or procedures. We encourage you to be creative and utilize the game model as an approach that has almost limitless variations and applications.

Group Game Programs

When leaders are using games as a method to address a particular goal or teach a specific skill, it is important to have a planned program. This program needs to be developed to reflect: (1) the mutual needs of the group members, (2) each individual's baseline knowledge and skills specific to the needs, and (3) the learning objectives or desired outcome of the group program.

Identification of needs and referrals for the focus of the group socialization programs can occur as a structured component of a habilitation or rehabilitation plan or on an as needed basis. For example, group programs that focus on commonly identified needs such as increasing prosocial behavior or developing effective coping and self-management skills may be scheduled at regular intervals (i.e., quarterly or semi-annually). Other referral concerns that are more situation-specific, such as conflict resolution, can be addressed when the need is identified.

We have found that group socialization programs are particularly helpful in assisting individuals in coping with adjustment to changes in work and living situations (i.e., competitive work and supported living). It becomes the challenge of the group planners to develop a program that responds to the referral concerns in an organized, individualized and outcome-based manner.

DEVELOPING THE PROGRAM

Depending on the availability of group members and leaders, planners must initially determine the number and length of sessions. Once that has been established, planners can then map out the sequential steps to obtain the desired outcome.

Based on the outcome focus, leaders must pay particular attention to facilitating learning and application of concepts by using specific design factors and specialized methods. Methods include beginning with basic concepts which are then reviewed and expanded in each successive session. In addition, games and activities are chosen and/or designed to reflect the groups specific theme or members' frame of reference. For example, if a group program is being developed for individuals who are experiencing problems getting along with peers at work, activities and games need to be chosen or developed that relate to work issues and environments. It is important for leaders to repeatedly focus members on the outcome and their progress to date throughout the group program.

Specific materials (i.e., folders, photos, handouts, graphics, etc.) can be used to concretize the steps towards reaching the group goal. We have found folders to be especially helpful for organizing information and providing memory cues for recall. Folders with weekly papers that visually or narratively describe activities and outcomes can be a very useful enhancement of the group program. Depending on the functional abilities of group members, leaders may provide varying degrees of assistance to support members paperwork. For individuals who have difficulty with generalization or applying learning from one situation to another, we have found support staff to be invaluable. They can assist members by cueing or reminding them of strategies learned and practiced in the group. They can also recognize and reinforce effective implementation of newly learned skills.

The group program outlines that follow consist of plans for six to eleven group sessions. The beginning sessions focus on basic aspects of self-awareness and then progress to social awareness and prosocial behaviors. Essential to designing a successful group program is meeting the individual members' needs for attention and focus on self. We attempt to structure time during each session for members to express themselves, or share information before beginning the structured group activity. The leader then facilitates a review of the previous session to promote ongoing awareness of the group focus and goals and continuity from session to session. The leader uses questioning and verbal prompts to cue the member's recall of the previous session so that they are actively involved in the review. For example, the leader may ask if members remember what they did or talked about the previous week or use a brief description of a specific situation or scenario from that session as a memory cue.

The specific games or structured activities included in each group program were chosen to address the needs and focus of our group members, but may be substituted with other similar games. Based on the group member's interests and abilities, the content, methods and pace may need to be adjusted or adapted. For example, during Basic Socialization Skills, Session #4, focusing on "How I Feel," the leader may encourage members to share recent personal situations and their related feelings. As much as possible, group leaders must attempt to make the connection between the group focus and content and the member's real-life experiences.

An important part of each group program should be evaluation based on group goals and desired outcomes. We have found that the most immediate and direct way to informally assess member's progress is by asking outcome-oriented "Yes—No" questions at the end of each session and at the end of the group program. For group members who demonstrate higher cognitive abilities, open-ended questions such as "What did you learn about _____?" or written assessments may be used. For sessions that focus on developing specific skills (i.e., anger management), members can be asked to demonstrate what they've learned. Support staff observations and reports can also provide important feedback related to member's progress. Although we do not routinely use formal evaluation methods (such as pre and post measures), we applaud leaders who are interested in the formal study of our methods.

GROUP PROGRAM OUTLINES

The following three outlines were designed to focus on developing basic social skills, positive work behaviors and interpersonal problem-solving skills.

Basic Socialization Group Program Outline

The basic social skills outline was developed for individuals who lived together and had limited personal involvement with each other. The group goal, or desired outcome was to help the individuals learn more about each others' positive characteristics and increase their prosocial interactions.

GOAL AREA	SESSION TOPICS AND ACTIVITIES
Self-Awareness	1. **Group Orientation**

    a) Member introductions.

    b) Review of group rules and goals.

    c) Leader takes each member's photograph. As photos are distributed, members are asked to share a special interest or positive characteristic.

    d) Leader discusses the group program outline and collects the photos for future sessions.

Self-Awareness	2.	**How I Look**

        a) Review of previous session.

        b) Members play the game "Name Warm-up."

        c) Members play the game "Looking at Myself," or leader hands out photographs and members take turns sharing things they like about their appearance.

        d) Leader collects photos for future sessions.

        e) Leader assists members with summarizing session.

Self-Awareness	3.	**Things I Like To Do**

        a) Review of previous session.

        b) Members take turns sharing "good things" or something positive they did during the week/day.

        c) Members play the game "Do you agree?" or members play "Guess What I'm Doing . . ."

        d) Leader assists members with summarizing sessions.

Self-Awareness	4.	**How I Feel**

        a) Review of previous session.

        b) Members take turns sharing something that made them feel good that day (or week).

        c) Members play "Happy, Sad or Mad" and discuss basic feeling states.

        d) If time permits, members may share personal experiences and related feelings.

        e) Leader assists members with summarizing session.

Self-Awareness	5.	**What I Do When I'm Angry**

        a) Review of previous session.

        b) Members take turns sharing a recent situation that made them feel mad/angry and how they responded.

        c) Leader asks the members to evaluate whether the response was "cool" or "OK," or "not cool." Other members are encouraged to give feedback.

d) Members play the game "Cool or Not."
e) Leader assists members with summarizing session.

Self-Awareness

6. **O.K. Ways to Show Anger**
   a) Review of previous session.
   b) Members take turns sharing their preferred "OK" ways of handling mad/angry feelings.
   c) Leader asks members to demonstrate their strategies and encourages other members to give feedback.
   d) Questions for discussion include: Has this worked for you? What happened? Tell us how it worked. If not, what happened? How did you feel? How did others feel? Would you change your way?
   e) Leader assists members with summarizing session.

Prosocial

7. **Special Friends**
   a) Review of previous session.
   b) Members take turns sharing information about a special friend (name, shared interests/activities/etc.).
   c) Members play "Do You Agree?" II.
   d) Members share personal stories about friends.
   e) Leader assists members with summarizing session.

Prosocial

8. **Helping Others**
   a) Review of previous session.
   b) Members take turns sharing something they've done to help another person recently or during the past week.
   c) Members play the game "Helping My Friend" I or "How Can I Help?"
   d) Leader assists members with summarizing session.

Prosocial

9. **Sharing With Others**
   a) Review previous session.
   b) Members take turns telling about a time they shared with another person.

c) Members play the game "Do I Care to Share?"
d) Leader assists members with summarizing session.

Prosocial   10. **Thinking About Other's Feelings**
a) Review of previous session.
b) Members take turns sharing something they did that made another person feel good/happy.
c) Members play the game "How I make others feel" or "Helping my friend feel good."
d) Leader assists members with summarizing session.

Self-Awareness   11. **Celebrating the Group**
a) Members play "Feelings About Our Group."
b) Members take turns sharing what they liked about the group and what changes, if any, they would make.
c) Members and leader(s) celebrate the relationships and group experience with a special snack or party.
d) Leader assists members with summarizing and evaluating the group.

Work Adjustment Group Program Outline

The work adjustment group outline was developed for individuals who were experiencing difficulties with the demands and expectations of competitive employment. The group goal and desired outcome was to assist in developing more socially acceptable behaviors in the work environment.

GOAL AREA   **SESSION TOPICS AND ACTIVITIES**
Self-Awareness   1. **Group Orientation**
a) Introduction—Review of group rules and goals as follows:
1. To learn about different job responsibilities.
2. To practice solving problems on-the-job.
b) Group members take turns telling about where they live and work.

   c) Group leader takes each member's photo and
      gives them a folder. In the folder is a list
      of session dates with the group goals. Each
      member can decorate or write on his/her
      folder. The folder is collected by the leader
      at the end of the session.
   e) Leader assists members with summarizing
      session.

Self-Awareness   2. **"Who Am I?"**
   a) Review previous week's session.
   b) Members play the game "Looking At Myself."
   c) Members play "Guess My Job," leader could
      write all jobs guessed on the blackboard/
      marker board for review purposes.
   e) Leader assists members with summarizing
      session.

Self-Awareness   3. **"Thinking About My Job"**
   a) Review previous week's session.
   b) Members play "Feeling Meter" with each
      member rating feelings about his/her present
      job. Leader reminds members that these
      feelings will be talked about again during
      later groups.
   c) Members play "What I Really Like About
      My Job."
   e) Leader assists members with summarizing
      session.

Self-Awareness   4. **Appearance On-the-job**
and Social
Competency
   a) Review previous week's session.
   b) Review each person's job by playing the game
      "Find the Person." Leader uses job list from
      session #2 instead of picture cards.
   c) Members play "Something's Wrong with
      Those Clothes."
   d) Group leader could videotape, if possible, for
      members to critique. (Alternate activity)
   e) Group leader facilitates discussion about
      appearance and hygiene at work. Members

may be given a piece of paper to write about or make a collage about items used for looking good at work. These papers could be shared with the group and then placed in their folders.

    f) Leader assists members with summarizing session.

Social Competency

5. **Accepting Supervision**
    a) Review previous session.
    b) Members play "Should I Ask for Help?"
    c) Members play "Don't Lose Your Cool II" (Related to work issues)
    d) Leader encourages members to share personal scenarios involving supervisors for discussion.
    e) Leader assists members with summarizing session.

Prosocial

6. **Co-Workers**
    a) Review previous session.
    b) Members play "Friendly or Not."
    c) Members play "I Like It When." (Related to co-workers).
    d) Leader assists members with summarizing session.

Social Competency

7. **Problem-Solving on the Job.**
    a) Review previous session.
    b) Members play "Whose Problem?"
    c) Members play "I Have a Problem. Can You Help?"
    d) Leader facilitates members sharing personal scenarios related to problems on the job. Then, members are encouraged to suggest solutions.
    e) Leader assists members with summarizing session.

Self-Awareness and Prosocial

8. **Problem-Solving on the Job.**
    a) Review previous session.
    b) Members play "Paying Attention to My Work."

c) Group members take turns sharing personal situations related to paying attention to the job.
d) Group begins to discuss what to do about feelings on-the-job or OK ways to handle their feelings at work.
e) Leader assists members with summarizing session.

Social Competency

9. **Behavior/Feelings and Self-Control**
   a) Review previous session.
   b) Members play "Keeping My Cool."
   c) Leaders demonstrate and members practice impulse control techniques such as counting to 10, deep breathing, or freezing in place.
   d) Leader assists members with writing down "My Way to Calm Down" and putting it in their folder.
   e) Leader assists members with summarizing session.

Social Awareness

10. **Review, Wrap-Up and Party**
    a) Review previous sessions; Leaders may hand out folders/photos for members to keep.
    b) Members play "We Had a Great Group!" or "I Know Something Good About. . . ."
    c) Snack, sharing, closure.
    d) Leader assists members with summarizing and evaluating the group.

Conflict Resolution Group Program Outline

The conflict resolution program outline was developed for use with groups of housemates and co-workers who were experiencing difficulties getting along with each other. The group goal or desired outcome was to assist in developing positive interpersonal connections, cooperative problem-solving skills, and a specific plan to resolve the identified conflicts.

GOAL AREA	SESSION TOPICS AND ACTIVITIES

Social Awareness 1. **What we have in common.**

    a) Introduction and facilitated discussion regarding the goals of the group as follows:
      1. To help us understand our needs.
      2. To work together to meet each of our needs.
      3. To feel better about each other.

    b) Members share previous positive experience together to establish a positive foundation for change. Members play "Remember When."

    c) Review and summarize positive events that members enjoyed with goal of increasing these experiences.

Self-Awareness 2. **What I need.**

    a) Review of previous session and group goals.

    b) Members play the game; "I Would Feel Better If _____." Members take turns responding to different aspects of their relationship as to whether it's OK or could be better.

    c) Leader assists members with summarizing session.

Social Competency 3. **Expressing my needs.**

    a) Review of previous session.

    b) Members play "What Works for Me."

    c) Each member is encouraged to talk about one important need that they have. i.e., privacy, space, help.

    d) Leader assists members with identifying ways to help each member meet his/her need.

    e) Leader assists members with summarizing session.

Social Competency 4. **Working out our problems.**

    a) Review of previous session. Discussion focuses on mutual needs and how to meet them.

    b) Members play "We All Win."

    c) Members discuss personal scenarios and are assisted in coming up with "winning" solutions for all.

      d) Leader assists members with summarizing sessions.

Social Competency 5.   **Making our plan.**

      a) Review of previous session.

      b) Continuing personal scenarios and problem-solving.

      c) Group development of conflict resolution plan. Plans include the agreed upon steps that each person will implement to resolve each problem. For example, if the problem is household tasks that are not completed consistently, then the plan would consist of each member's specific responsibilities to complete the task. (Additional follow-up sessions are recommended for review of the group's progress related to the plan or to focus on "How We're Doing").

      d) Leader facilitates members' recognition of one another for successful development of the plan and members all shake hands.

      e) Leader assists members with summarizing progress towards ongoing goals/outcomes.

SECTION 5

SOCIALIZATION GAMES

This section describes more than 100 socialization games and outlines the materials and procedures for playing each game. The games are arranged in terms of five socialization areas: interpersonal distance, self-awareness, social awareness, prosocial behavior, and social competence. They are coded in terms of a game assessment scheme to indicate the competencies that are required of the participants, the focus of rewards, the degree of psychological risk-taking, and group involvement, whether the game is appropriate for the beginning, the middle or the closing sessions of group life, and the amount of preparation time and materials that are necessary.

THE GAME ASSESSMENT SCHEME

The game assessment scheme* is designed to help the leader make a match between the requirements of a game and the characteristics of the group. To select a game, one scans the left margin of the assessment scheme to note the features. A group leader should examine and compare the characteristics of group members with each game feature that is being considered. For example, when examining the feature of "functional competencies" the group leader may informally assess his/her group members in terms of their level of communication. If many members have difficulty in expressive communication, then a game that is low in this feature should be chosen. Thus, the game assessment scheme is a guide for making a decision about whether a specific game should be used with a particular group.

While it is easier to select games for a more homogeneous group, or a group in which members have similar skill levels, one may not have the opportunity of working with such a group. To provide for the interest

---

*A prototype of the assessment scheme was used by Bendekovic (1971) in comparing and contrasting an array of structured group activities.

and success of all members of a heterogeneous group requires planning and thoughtful selection of game activities by the leader. A workable approach at times is to select games based on the abilities of the less skilled individuals and provide for the higher skilled individuals by giving them assisting roles and the opportunity to expand or elaborate the procedures. For example, in the game "I Wish," less-skilled individuals may identify concrete objects whereas higher skilled individuals may be encouraged to express dreams or fantasies.

At other times one can select games requiring slightly more complex skills and, again, the higher skilled members would be encouraged to assist the lower skilled members through the game activity. For example, in the game "Where Is the Button?" lower skilled individuals in some of our groups were able to recognize the button, but were often unable to think of a good hiding place, or, to look for the button with a systematic approach. Higher skilled individuals were asked to help these members hide the button in less visible places; and escort them around the group to demonstrate a systematic approach.

Six primary features are identified via the game assessment scheme: (1) socialization area, (2) competence needed, (3) focus of rewards, (4) psychological risks, (5) group aspects, and (6) administration. Each of these features and their sub-characteristics are discussed below.

1. *Socialization Area.* This term refers to the goal of each game. Some games have more than one socialization purpose, but they are described in terms of the goal that seems primary.

2. *Competence Needed.* This is a term for the skills that are required of participants. These include the levels of communication, motor behavior, and cognition that individuals need in order to participate successfully in the game.

   Communication. *Low* communication games can be played by group members who have limited expressive abilities. *High* communication games require that most members be able to communicate effectively with others in the group. The game "Do This" is low in communication as is "Stare Down," because they require only motor imitation. The game "I Like You Because . . . " is high in communication because it requires members to state what they like about other group members.

   Motor Behavior. Some games can be utilized with people who have limited motor abilities. *High* motor games require group members to leave their seats and move about. "Who's Talking" is a low motor game as group members sit and listen to a tape recorder and try to guess which group member is talking. In "We Have A Lot in Common," members must move from station to station as various characteristics or attributes are named by the leader. For example, everyone wearing glasses is told to move to a specific area in the room.

Cognitive Requirement. This feature refers to the cognitive skills required by the game. While cognitive requirement is related to rule complexity and conceptual abilities, it specifically refers to the complexity of the behavior required by the games. Low cognitive requirement games involve only simple imitation. Games *high* in cognitive requirement may involve role play, modeling or analysis of a problem and generation of solutions. "Beat the Buzzer" places a low cognitive demand on members as they are only required to put a hat and mittens on another member and members may learn how to perform by imitation. "What Am I Doing" is a high cognitive demand game because members must enact situations and problem solve.

3. *Focus of Rewards.* The group procedure suggested in Section 3 emphasizes that social recognition be provided throughout the group session. However, the games vary in terms of the focus of rewards that are suggested. Some games provide rewards to individual participants. Other games provide rewards to all group members at the same time. As an incentive for certain individuals, leaders may want to select a game that provides tangible rewards to individuals. However, in order to develop group spirit the leader may choose a game in which rewards are provided contingent upon the group's performance. The "to whom" dimension of the reward feature shows whether the reward goes to an *individual* or to the *group.* The reward feature of "Blow Round" is a tangible payoff to the group. If group members can maintain a ping pong ball on a table top by blowing it away from the edge for a specified time period, e.g., one minute, then all group members receive a snack. Alternatively, other games such as "I Have a Problem— How Can You Help?" provide for individual rewards. The member with the problem and the member who provides the solution are recognized individually for their efforts.

4. *Psychological Risks.* Leaders experienced in group work realize that group participation may expose members to criticism, embarrassment, or ridicule from others. Some of the games ask members to disclose their feelings, preferences, and wishes. The psychological risk factor inherent in self-disclosure may make some group members uncomfortable when initially playing some games. Games that require no self-disclosure are labelled *low,* and those which do call for self-disclosure are labelled *high* risk. "Find the Person" is low in psychological risk because members are not asked to reveal personal information. "Let Me Tell You How I'm Feeling Today" is a game high in psychological risk because group members are asked to disclose and share how they feel about certain situations.

5. *Group Aspects.* Group aspects consists of two dimensions, *involvement* and *phase of group development.*

Involvement. This is the extent to which the game promotes simultaneous involvement of all group members or, conversely, involves only one or two members at a time. *Low* involvement means that one or two members are active at a time. *High* involvement means that all or most group members are involved at one time. "Blow Round" is an example of a high involvement game.

Phases of Group Development. This dimension indicates whether a game is appropriate for the *warm-up phase,* the *game (main) phase,* or the *closing phase* of group life as explained in Section 3. During the warm-up phase, the leader is focusing primarily on teaching members to maintain attention, follow directions, respect rules and take turns. Games appropriate for the warm-up phase are usually action-oriented, simple, and *high* in member involvement. These games promote interest and enthusiasm in the group while helping the members develop basic group skills. Games/activities appropriate for the game phase, generally, place more cognitive demand on members and may be less action-oriented. Lastly, the games that are appropriate for the closing phase of the group alert members to the approaching completion of the group program and allow them to gain closure to the group experience. This dimension enables a group leader to select games that he/she feels are appropriate to the phase of group life.

6. *Administration.* Group leaders may not have access to funds to secure supplies or time to invest in lengthy preparation and plan-

ning for a group session. Two features, *materials* and *preparation/planning,* have been included to facilitate game selection.

Materials. The supplies that are needed are listed on each game sheet under "materials." Games *low* in materials require few props. "Find Your Friend" is an example of a game which is low on this dimension. The game requires only a blindfold in addition to the standard set of photos* of group members. Games that are *high* in materials require a number of props or materials. For instance, the game "Mix or Match II" requires a number of personal or household articles.

Preparation/Planning. This refers to the amount of preparation required. Planning and preparation can involve planning for role play situations, making stimulus cards, or obtaining props and other materials. *Low* planning and preparation means that little time is required in order to implement the game. The game "Back to Back" requires no props and little preparation and planning. *High* planning and preparation means that the leader must spend some time developing materials or planning specific problem situations, role plays or scenarios to implement the game. An example of a game demanding high planning and preparation is "Find the Person," as the materials include stimulus cards.

---

*A set of photographs of group members is used in many games and is an initial expense which is not considered in the rating of a game as either low or high with respect to the *materials* feature.

GAME ASSESSMENT SCHEME #1						
GAME TITLE	Blow Round	Do This	Don't Drop The Can	Guess Who? I	Hidden Object	I Wish
SOCIALIZATION GOALS	Inter-personal Distance	Inter-personal Distance	Inter-personal Distance	Inter-personal Distance	Inter-personal Distance	Inter-personal Distance
COMPETENCE NEEDED Expressive Communication	Low	Low	Low	Low	High	High
Motor	High	High	High	High	Low	Low
Cognitive Requirements	Low	Low	Low	Low	High	High
FOCUS OF REWARDS	Group	Group	Individual	Individual	Individual	Group
PSYCHOLOGICAL RISK	Low	Low	Low	Low	Low	High
GROUP ASPECTS Involvement	High	High	Low	Low	High	High
Phases of Group Development	Warm-up	Warm-up	Warm-up	Warm-up and Game Phase	Game Phase	Game Phase
ADMINISTRATION Materials	Low	Low	Low	Low	High	Low
Preparation & Planning	Low	Low	Low	Low	High	Low

GAME ASSESSMENT SCHEME #2						
GAME TITLE	Pass It Along	Working Together	Make Me Laugh	Mystery Object	Shape Match	Stare Down
SOCIALIZATION GOALS	Inter-personal Distance	Inter-personal Distance	Inter-personal Distance	Inter-personal Distance	Inter-personal Distance	Inter-personal Distance
COMPETENCE NEEDED Communication	Low	Low	Low	Low	Low	Low
Motor	High	High	Low	Low	High	Low
Cognitive Requirements	Low	Low	High	Low	Low	High
FOCUS OF REWARDS	Group	Individual	Individual	Individual	Individual	Individual
PSYCHOLOGICAL RISK	Low	Low	High	Low	Low	Low
GROUP ASPECTS Involvement	High	Low	Low	Low	High	Low
Phases of Group Development	Warm-up	Warm-up	Warm-up	Game Phase	Game Phase	Warm-up and Game Phase
ADMINISTRATION Materials	Low	Low	Low	High	High	Low
Preparation & Planning	Low	Low	Low	High	High	Low

GAME ASSESSMENT SCHEME #3						
GAME TITLE	Beat The Buzzer	Where's The Button?	Which Hand?	Working Together To Beat The Clock	Are You Happy or Are You Mad?	Feelings About Our Group
SOCIALIZATION GOALS	Inter-Personal Distance	Inter-Personal Distance	Inter-Personal Distance	Inter-Personal Distance	Self-Awareness	Self-Awareness
COMPETENCE NEEDED Communication	Low	Low	Low	Low	Low	Low
Motor	High (Upper Body)	High	High	High (Upper Body)	Low	Low
Cognitive Requirements	Low	High	High	Low	High	High
FOCUS OF REWARDS	Individual	Individual	Individual	Group	Individual	Individual
PSYCHOLOGICAL RISK	Low	Low	Low	Low	High	High
GROUP ASPECTS Involvement	High	High	Low	High	High	Low
Phases of Group Development	Warm-up	Warm-up and Game Phase	Game Phase	Warm-up	Game Phase	Termina-tion
ADMINISTRATION Materials	Low	Low	Low	High	High	High
Preparation & Planning	Low	Low	Low	High	High	High

GAME ASSESSMENT SCHEME #4						
GAME TITLE	Finish The Sentence	Here's How I'm Feeling Today	Signal If You Know I	I Feel Really Good About . . .	My Favorite Things	Name Warm-up
SOCIALIZATION GOALS	Self-Awareness	Self-Awareness	Self-Awareness	Self-Awareness	Self-Awareness	Self-Awareness
COMPETENCE NEEDED Communication	High	Low	High	High	High	High
Motor	Low	High	Low	Low	Low	Low
Cognitive Requirements	High	High	High	High	High	High
FOCUS OF REWARDS	Individual	Individual	Individual	Individual	Group	Individual
PSYCHOLOGICAL RISK	High	High	High	High	High	High
GROUP ASPECTS Involvement	Low	Low	Low	Low	Low	Low
Phases of Group Development	Game Phase	Game Phase	Game Phase	Game Phase	Game Phase	Warm-up Phase
ADMINISTRATION Materials	Low	Low	Low	Low	Low	Low
Preparation & Planning	Low	Low	Low	High	Low	Low

GAME ASSESSMENT SCHEME #5						
GAME TITLE	The Feeling Meter	Things We Like To Do Together	Do You Agree? I	Remember When	Happy, Sad or Mad	I Would Feel Better If
SOCIALIZATION GOALS	Self-Awareness	Self-Awareness	Self-Awareness	Self-Awareness	Self-Awareness	Self-Awareness
COMPETENCE NEEDED Communication	High	Low	High	High	Low	High
Motor	Low	Low	Low	Low	Low	Low
Cognitive Requirements	High	Low	High	High	Low	High
FOCUS OF REWARDS	Individual	Individual	Individual	Individual	Individual	Individual
PSYCHOLOGICAL RISK	High	Low	Low	Low	Low	High
GROUP ASPECTS Involvement	Low	High	High	High	High	Low
Phases of Group Development	Game Phase	Termination Phase	Game Phase	Game Phase	Game Phase	Game Phase
ADMINISTRATION Materials	High	High	High	High	High	High
Preparation & Planning	High	High	Low	High	Low	High

GAME ASSESSMENT SCHEME #6						
GAME TITLE	I Blew It	Guess What I'm Doing?	I Like It When	Telling About Myself	Paycheck Goes Up; Paycheck Goes Down	Paying Attention To My Work
SOCIALIZATION GOALS	Self-Awareness	Self-Awareness	Self-Awareness	Self-Awareness	Self-Awareness	Self-Awareness
COMPETENCE NEEDED Communication	High	Low	High	Low	Low	Low
Motor	Low	High	Low	Low	Low	Low
Cognitive Requirements	High	Low	High	Low	Low	High
FOCUS OF REWARDS	Individual	Group	Individual	Individual	Group	Group
PSYCHOLOGICAL RISK	High	Low	High	High	Low	Low
GROUP ASPECTS Involvement	High	High	High	Low	High	High
Phases of Group Development	Game Phase	Warm-up Phase	Game Phase	Warm-up Phase	Game Phase	Game Phase
ADMINISTRATION Materials	Low	Low	Low	High	Low	Low
Preparation & Planning	Low	Low	Low	Low	High	High

GAME ASSESSMENT SCHEME #7						
GAME TITLE	What I Really Like About My Job	Been There, Done That	Like It or Not	What's Missing?	It's OK By Me or I Want To Make A Change	Back To Back
SOCIALIZATION GOALS	Self-Awareness	Self-Awareness	Self-Awareness	Self-Awareness	Self-Awareness	Social Awareness
COMPETENCE NEEDED Communication	High	Low	Low	Low	High	High
Motor	Low	Low	Low	Low	Low	Low
Cognitive Requirements	High	High	Low	Low	High	High
FOCUS OF REWARDS	Group	Group	Group	Individual	Individual	Individual
PSYCHOLOGICAL RISK	High	Low	Low	Low	High	Low
GROUP ASPECTS Involvement	High	High	High	High	Low	Low
Phases of Group Development	Game Phase	Game Phase	Game Phase	Game Phase	Game Phase	Game Phase
ADMINISTRATION Materials	Low	High	High	High	Low	Low
Preparation & Planning	Low	High	High	Low	High	Low

GAME ASSESSMENT SCHEME #8						
GAME TITLE	Can You Pretend?	Clothing Color Match	Find The Owner	Find Your Friend	Find The Person	Signal If You Know II
SOCIALIZATION GOALS	Social Awareness	Social Awareness	Social Awareness	Social Awareness	Social Awareness	Social Awareness
COMPETENCE NEEDED Communication	Low	Low	Low	Low	Low	High
Motor	High	High	High	High	High	Low
Cognitive Requirements	High	Low	High	Low	Low	High
FOCUS OF REWARDS	Individual	Individual	Individual	Individual	Individual	Individual
PSYCHOLOGICAL RISK	High	Low	Low	Low	Low	High
GROUP ASPECTS Involvement	High	Low	Low	High	Low	High
Phases of Group Development	Game Phase	Game Phase	Game Phase	Game Phase	Game Phase	Game Phase
ADMINISTRATION Materials	Low	High	High	Low	High	Low
Preparation & Planning	Low	High	High	Low	High	Low

GAME ASSESSMENT SCHEME #9						
GAME TITLE	I Know Something About You	If I Were You	Name Draw	Name Game I	Name Game II	Pick A Friend
SOCIALIZATION GOALS	Social Awareness	Social Awareness	Social Awareness	Social Awareness	Social Awareness	Social Awareness
COMPETENCE NEEDED Communication	High	Low	High	Low	Low	High
Motor	Low	High	High	High	High	Low
Cognitive Requirements	High	High	High	Low	Low	High
FOCUS OF REWARDS	Individual	Individual	Individual	Group	Group	Individual
PSYCHOLOGICAL RISK	Low	Low	Low	Low	Low	Low
GROUP ASPECTS Involvement	Low	Low	Low	High	High	High
Phases of Group Development	Game Phase	Game Phase	Warm-up Phase	Warm-up Phase	Warm-up Phase	Game Phase
ADMINISTRATION Materials	Low	Low	Low	Low	Low	Low
Preparation & Planning	Low	Low	Low	Low	Low	Low

GAME ASSESSMENT SCHEME #10						
GAME TITLE	Seeing The Best	The Blindfold Game	TV Star	We Had A Great Group!	We Have A Lot in Common	Whisper
SOCIALIZATION GOALS	Social Awareness	Social Awareness	Social Awareness	Social Awareness	Social Awareness	Social Awareness
COMPETENCE NEEDED Communication	Low	Low	High	Low	Low	Low
Motor	Low	Low	Low	Low	High	High
Cognitive Requirements	High	Low	High	High	Low	Low
FOCUS OF REWARDS	Individual	Individual	Individual	Individual	Group	Individual
PSYCHOLOGICAL RISK	Low	Low	Low	Low	High	Low
GROUP ASPECTS Involvement	Low	Low	High	High	High	Low
Phases of Group Development	Game Phase	Game Phase	Game Phase	Termination Phase	Game Phase	Game Phase
ADMINISTRATION Materials	Low	Low	High	High	Low	Low
Preparation & Planning	Low	Low	High	High	Low	Low

GAME ASSESSMENT SCHEME #11						
GAME TITLE	Who Am I Talking About?	Who Is This Person?	Who's Missing?	Guess Who? II	I Know Something Good About	Guess My Job
SOCIALIZATION GOALS	Social Awareness	Social Awareness	Social Awareness	Social Awareness	Social Awareness	Social Awareness
COMPETENCE NEEDED Communication	High	Low	Low	High	High	Low
Motor	Low	Low	Low	Low	Low	High
Cognitive Requirements	High	Low	High	High	High	Low
FOCUS OF REWARDS	Group	Group	Individual	Individual	Individual	Individual
PSYCHOLOGICAL RISK	Low	Low	Low	Low	High	Low
GROUP ASPECTS Involvement	Low	High	High	High	High	Low
Phases of Group Development	Game Phase	Game Phase	Game Phase	Game Phase	Game Phase	Game Phase
ADMINISTRATION Materials	Low	Low	Low	High	Low	Low
Preparation & Planning	Low	Low	Low	High	High	Low

GAME ASSESSMENT SCHEME #12						
GAME TITLE	Birthday Box	Do You Agree? II	Good For You	Friendship Chain	Helping Each Other	Helping My Friend Find His/ Her Stuff
SOCIALIZATION GOALS	Social Awareness	Social Awareness	Social Awareness	Prosocial	Prosocial	Prosocial
COMPETENCE NEEDED Communication	Low	Low	High	High	Low	Low
Motor	Low	Low	Low	High	High	High
Cognitive Requirements	Low	High	High	High	Low	Low
FOCUS OF REWARDS	Individual	Group	Individual	Individual	Individual	Individual
PSYCHOLOGICAL RISK	Low	High	High	High	Low	Low
GROUP ASPECTS Involvement	High	High	High	High	Low	High
Phases of Group Development	Game Phase	Game Phase	Game Phase	Game Phase	Game Phase	Game Phase
ADMINISTRATION Materials	High	Low	Low	Low	High	High
Preparation & Planning	High	Low	High	Low	High	High

GAME ASSESSMENT SCHEME #13						
GAME TITLE	Helping My Friend I	Helping My Friend II	I Have A Problem. How Can You Help?	The Magic Box I	The Magic Box II	Do I Care to Share?
SOCIALIZATION GOALS	Prosocial	Prosocial	Prosocial	Prosocial	Prosocial	Prosocial
COMPETENCE NEEDED Communication	Low	High	Low	Low	Low	Low
Motor	High	Low	High	Low	High	Low
Cognitive Requirements	Low	High	High	Low	High	High
FOCUS OF REWARDS	Individual	Individual	Individual	Individual	Individual	Individual
PSYCHOLOGICAL RISK	Low	High	Low	Low	High	High
GROUP ASPECTS Involvement	High	High	Low	Low	Low	Low
Phases of Group Development	Game Phase	Game Phase	Game Phase	Game Phase	Game Phase	Game Phase
ADMINISTRATION Materials	High	Low	Low	High	High	Low
Preparation & Planning	High	Low	Low	High	High	Low

GAME ASSESSMENT SCHEME #14						
GAME TITLE	How Others Feel	Helping Others Feel Good	Friendly or Not	I Have a Problem. How Can You Help? II	What Am I Doing?	Good Times We Shared
SOCIALIZATION GOALS	Prosocial	Prosocial	Prosocial	Prosocial	Prosocial	Prosocial
COMPETENCE NEEDED Communication	High	High	Low	High	Low	High
Motor	Low	Low	Low	Low	High	Low
Cognitive Requirements	High	High	High	High	Low	High
FOCUS OF REWARDS	Individual	Individual	Group	Individual	Individual	Individual
PSYCHOLOGICAL RISK	High	High	Low	High	High	High
GROUP ASPECTS Involvement	High	High	High	Low	Low	Low
Phases of Group Development	Game Phase	Game Phase	Game Phase	Game Phase	Game Phase	Game Phase
ADMINISTRATION Materials	Low	Low	Low	Low	Low	Low
Preparation & Planning	High	High	Low	Low	Low	High

GAME ASSESSMENT SCHEME #15						
GAME TITLE	What Works For Me	We All Win	Doin' The Spring Thing	Being Responsible I	Being Responsible II	Don't Lose Your Cool I
SOCIALIZATION GOALS	Prosocial	Prosocial	Prosocial	Social Competence	Social Competence	Social Competence
COMPETENCE NEEDED Communication	High	High	Low	Low	High	Low
Motor	Low	Low	High	Low	Low	Low
Cognitive Requirements	High	High	Low	High	High	Low
FOCUS OF REWARDS	Individual	Group	Individual	Group	Individual	Individual
PSYCHOLOGICAL RISK	High	High	Low	High	High	High
GROUP ASPECTS Involvement	Low	High	High	High	Low	High
Phases of Group Development	Game Phase	Game Phase	Game Phase	Game Phase	Game Phase	Game Phase
ADMINISTRATION Materials	Low	Low	Low	High	Low	Low
Preparation & Planning	Low	High	Low	High	High	Low

GAME ASSESSMENT SCHEME #16						
GAME TITLE	Don't Lose Your Cool II	Mix and Match I	Weather Match	Should I Ask For Help?	Something's Wrong With Those Clothes!	The Greeting Game
SOCIALIZATION GOALS	Social Compe-tence	Social Compe-tence	Social Compe-tence	Social Compe-tence	Social Compe-tence	Social Compe-tence
COMPETENCE NEEDED Communication	High	Low	Low	Low	Low	Low
Motor	Low	High	High	Low	High	High
Cognitive Requirements	High	High	High	High	High	High
FOCUS OF REWARDS	Individual	Individual	Individual	Individual	Individual	Individual
PSYCHOLOGICAL RISK	High	Low	Low	High	Low	High
GROUP ASPECTS Involvement	High	High	High	High	Low	High
Phases of Group Development	Game Phase	Game Phase	Game Phase	Game Phase	Game Phase	Game Phase
ADMINISTRATION Materials	Low	High	High	High	High	Low
Preparation & Planning	Low	High	High	High	High	High

GAME ASSESSMENT SCHEME #17						
GAME TITLE	Mix and Match II	Who Can Help?	Mix and Match III	Whose Problem?	Finding My Way	Thumbs Up or Thumbs Down I
SOCIALIZATION GOALS	Social Compe-tence	Social Compe-tence	Social Compe-tence	Social Compe-tence	Social Compe-tence	Social Compe-tence
COMPETENCE NEEDED Communication	Low	Low	Low	Low	High	Low
Motor	High	Low	Low	Low	Low	Low
Cognitive Requirements	High	High	High	High	High	High
FOCUS OF REWARDS	Individual	Individual	Individual	Individual	Individual	Group
PSYCHOLOGICAL RISK	Low	Low	High	High	High	High
GROUP ASPECTS Involvement	High	Low	High	Low	Low	High
Phases of Group Development	Game Phase	Game Phase	Game Phase	Game Phase	Game Phase	Game Phase
ADMINISTRATION Materials	High	High	High	Low	Low	Low
Preparation & Planning	High	High	High	Low	Low	Low

GAME ASSESSMENT SCHEME #18						
GAME TITLE	Thumbs Up Or Thumbs Down II	What Would You Do?	OK or No Way	You're The Boss	Stop and Think	What Works For Me When I'm Sad
SOCIALIZATION GOALS	Social Compe-tence	Social Compe-tence	Social Compe-tence	Social Compe-tence	Social Compe-tence	Social Compe-tence
COMPETENCE NEEDED Communication	Low	High	Low	High	Low	High
Motor	Low	Low	High	Low	Low	High
Cognitive Requirements	High	High	High	High	High	High
FOCUS OF REWARDS	Group	Individual	Group	Individual	Group	Individual
PSYCHOLOGICAL RISK	High	High	Low	High	Low	High
GROUP ASPECTS Involvement	High	High	High	Low	High	High
Phases of Group Development	Game Phase	Game Phase	Game Phase	Game Phase	Game Phase	Game Phase
ADMINISTRATION Materials	Low	Low	Low	Low	Low	Low
Preparation & Planning	Low	Low	High	High	High	High

GAME ASSESSMENT SCHEME #19					
GAME TITLE	What Works For Me When I'm Mad	Please Don't Tease I	Please Don't Tease II	Polite Or Not Right	Would This Person Be A Good Friend?
SOCIALIZATION GOALS	Social Competence	Social Competence	Social Competence	Social Competence	Social Competence
COMPETENCE NEEDED Communication	High	High	High	High	High
Motor	Low	Low	Low	Low	Low
Cognitive Requirements	High	High	High	High	High
FOCUS OF REWARDS	Individual	Group	Group	Individual	Group
PSYCHOLOGICAL RISK	High	High	High	Low	High
GROUP ASPECTS Involvement	High	High	High	High	High
Phases of Group Development	Game Phase	Game Phase	Game Phase	Game Phase	Game Phase
ADMINISTRATION Materials	Low	Low	Low	Low	Low
Preparation & Planning	High	High	High	High	High

INTERPERSONAL DISTANCE
LEARNING TO BE CLOSE TO OTHERS

"Blow Round"
"Do This . . ."
"Don't Drop The Can"
"Guess Who" I
"Hidden Object"
"I Wish"
"Pass It Along"
"Working Together"
"Make Me Laugh"
"Mystery Object"
"Shape Match"
"Stare Down"
"Beat The Buzzer"
"Where's The Button?"
"Which Hand?"
"Working Together To Beat The Clock"

TITLE: **"Blow Round"**

SOCIALIZATION
GOAL AREA: Interpersonal Distance/Learning to be Close to Others

MATERIALS: Table, chairs, ping pong ball, pretzels

GAME PROCEDURE: Group members are seated around the table and instructed to place their chins close to the table. The leader then rolls a ping pong ball onto the table and tells the members to try to blow it over to the other side of the table.* Throughout the game, members are told to keep the ball in motion. If the group is able to keep the ball on the table until the timer buzzes, all members are awarded snacks.

PARTICIPATION
PROCEDURE: Everyone in the group has a chance to participate at the same time.

SUGGESTIONS: One way to develop group cohesion is to gradually increase the length of time required for the reward.

TITLE: **"Do This . . . "**

SOCIALIZATION
GOAL AREA: Interpersonal Distance/Learning to be Close to Others

MATERIALS: No special materials needed

GAME PROCEDURE: Members are introduced to the cue "Do This" which means to imitate the behavior of the leader (in the fashion of "Simon Says"). The participants are instructed by the leader to "Do what I do when I say 'Do This'." Types of imitative responses that can be used in this game follow:

1) Body level of imitation: identifying/ touching body parts, e.g., touching head, nose, mouth.

---

*A timer is set for 30 seconds.

2) Verbal/sound level of imitation: vocalizations or verbalizations e.g., yodeling, singing, funny phrases.

3) Feeling level of imitation: mood and feelings, e.g., anger, sadness, happiness.

PARTICIPATION
PROCEDURE: Everyone in group has a chance to participate at the same time.

SUGGESTIONS: The leader may want to ask group members to take turns being the leader for a round of "Do This." It is possible that the member may have to be prompted in providing a response to be imitated. To do this, the leader may whisper a suggestion to the leader of the round.

TITLE: "Don't Drop The Can"

SOCIALIZATION
GOAL AREA: Interpersonal Distance/Learning to be Close to Others

MATERIALS: Coffee can, board that is approximately 3 feet long and 4 inches wide

GAME PROCEDURE: Starting and finishing points are marked on the floor with masking tape or objects.* Two group members are placed at the starting point and each given an end of the board with the coffee can placed in the center. The members are asked to help each other take the can to the finish line without dropping it. If members are able to get to the finish marker with no more than one drop of the can, special recognition is provided.

PARTICIPATION
PROCEDURE: Two members at a time are selected by the BLIND SELECTION METHOD.

---

*Approximately 25 feet apart.

SELECTION: To make the game more challenging the leader can partially fill the can with water.

TITLE: **"Guess Who?" I**

SOCIALIZATION
GOAL AREA: Interpersonal Distance/Learning To Be Close To Others

MATERIALS: No special materials are required.

GAME PROCEDURE: One member sits with his/her back to the group. The group members are seated in a semi-circle. Another member quietly walks up behind the seated member and puts hands over his/her eyes asking "Guess Who?" The seated member then must guess who is behind him/her.

PARTICIPATION
PROCEDURE: The BLIND SELECTION METHOD is used.

TITLE: **"Hidden Object"**

SOCIALIZATION
GOAL AREA: Interpersonal Distance/Learning to be Close to Others

MATERIALS: Small box, blindfold, familiar items (at least 1 per member) (see "Mystery Object")

GAME PROCEDURE: One member is blindfolded. Another member takes an object and hides it under a small box. The blindfold is removed and the member must guess what the object is with clues provided by the other members. Leaders can prompt group with questions like: What color is it?, How big is it?, Do you wear it?, Where do you keep it?, What do you do with it?, etc.

PARTICIPATION
PROCEDURE: The BLIND SELECTION METHOD is used with the member hiding the object becoming the next to be blindfolded.

TITLE: **"I Wish"**

SOCIALIZATION
GOAL AREA: Interpersonal Distance/Learning to be Close to Others

MATERIALS: No special materials are required

GAME PROCEDURE: A member thinks of a wish (with assistance from the leader, if needed). The member whispers it to the person next to him/her and he/she passes it on. The wish is passed on until it gets to the person seated next to the one who started it. This person then announces the wish to the group. The person who started it then tells his/her wish to the group.

PARTICIPATION
PROCEDURE: Group members can take turns in order or the BLIND SELECTION METHOD can be used.

SUGGESTIONS: The leader may have to act as a "bridge" in getting a message from one group member to another. However, the leader should only intervene when a group member is having difficulty in attending or has communication problems.

TITLE: **"Pass It Along"**

SOCIALIZATION
GOAL AREA: Interpersonal Distance/Learning to be Close to Others

MATERIALS: No special materials are required

GAME PROCEDURE: The leader imitates a gross motor act to the group member on his/her right (arm waving, tapping head, clapping hands, etc.). The member is instructed to pass the act to his/her right, with each member continuing to pass the act until it comes back to the leader. The group members rate whether or not the final act matches the original act. The member to the right of the leader is then instructed to pass his/her own different act around the circle.

PARTICIPATION
PROCEDURE: The LEADER SELECTION METHOD is used, until all have had a turn.

TITLE: **"Working Together"**

SOCIALIZATION
GOAL AREA: Interpersonal Distance/Learning to be Close to Others

MATERIALS: Ball, orange or similar object

GAME PROCEDURE: Starting and finishing points are marked on the floor with tape or objects.* Two members are told that a ball, orange, or similar object will be placed between their arms and that they must help each other by holding their arms tightly together. The members are instructed to walk from the start to the finish marker without dropping the ball, orange, or similar object. If members are able to reach the finish line with no more than one drop, they receive special recognition.

PARTICIPATION
PROCEDURE: Two members at a time are selected by the BLIND SELECTION METHOD.

TITLE: **"Make Me Laugh"**

SOCIALIZATION
GOAL AREA: Interpersonal Distance/Learning to be Close to Others

MATERIALS: No special materials are required

GAME PROCEDURE: Two group members sit across from one another. One group member takes the role of "acting silly." The "silly" member makes a face

---

*Placed approximately 25 feet apart.

or a funny movement and attempts to make his partner "crack up" (laugh). The partner tries to keep from laughing. However, when the partner does laugh, the members switch roles.

PARTICIPATION
PROCEDURE: Two group members at a time are selected by the BLIND SELECTION METHOD.

SUGGESTIONS: The group member who is taking the role of "being silly" may need prompts to make the other laugh. The leader can go through a three step procedure of prompts. First, the leader can say to the member, "Make a funny face." If this doesn't work, the leader should try a concrete verbal suggestion like "Make a face like a monkey." Finally, if this doesn't work, the leader can model a funny face to the member and ask him/her to imitate it.

TITLE: **"Mystery Object"**

SOCIALIZATION
GOAL AREA: Interpersonal Distance/Learning to be Close to Others

MATERIALS: Box of familiar objects, e.g., brush, scissors, spoon, cup, glasses, toothbrush, and a blindfold.

GAME PROCEDURE: One member is blindfolded. Another member selects an item from the box and presents it to the blindfolded member for identification. Clues as to the use of the object may serve as prompts.

PARTICIPATION
PROCEDURE: The BLIND SELECTION METHOD is used to select group members. The member presenting the object then becomes the next blindfolded member.

TITLE: **"Shape Match"**

SOCIALIZATION
GOAL AREA: Interpersonal Distance/Learning to be Close to Others

MATERIALS: Two small boxes or containers, two sets of matching shapes, e.g., circle, triangle, square, cross, heart, star, diamond, etc., blindfold

GAME PROCEDURE: Each set of shapes is put into a box or small container. Each member selects a shape from one box. One member is blindfolded and draws a shape from the matching shape box. The member must then find the group member with the matching shape.

PARTICIPATION
PROCEDURE: The BLIND SELECTION METHOD is used to select group members. The matching member then becomes the next member to be blindfolded.

TITLE: **"Stare Down"**

SOCIALIZATION
GOAL AREA: Interpersonal Distance/Learning to be Close to Others

MATERIALS: No special materials are required

GAME PROCEDURE: Two group members sit facing one another. Both members are instructed to "stare" at the other member, and to keep from "cracking up"—that is, keep from laughing. The member who refrains from laughing (who stares the longest) wins the round. This member is then challenged by another member.

PARTICIPATION
PROCEDURE: For the first round, two members are chosen by the BLIND SELECTION METHOD. Thereafter, one member is chosen through the BLIND SELECTION METHOD to challenge the winner of each round.

TITLE: **"Beat the Buzzer"**

SOCIALIZATION
GOAL AREA: Interpersonal Distance/Learning to be Close to Others

MATERIALS: 2 hats, 2 pairs of mittens and Kitchen Timer

GAME PROCEDURE: Two members sit facing each other in the center of the group. Both are given a hat and mittens and instructed to "put them on your partner." If all items are on before the bell rings, each member receives special recognition.

PARTICIPATION
PROCEDURE: The BLIND SELECTION METHOD is used until all members have had a turn.

TITLE: **"Where's the Button?"**

SOCIALIZATION
GOAL AREA: Interpersonal Distance/Learning to be Close to Others

MATERIALS: 1 paper "button" (a circle approximately $\frac{1}{2}''$ in diameter) with adhesive tape on the back, blindfold

GAME PROCEDURE: Group members are shown the "button" and told that they will each have a turn to hide the button on another group member. One member is blindfolded and another member hides the button by placing it on a member's person. Members are encouraged to find a different place to hide it each time. The blindfold is removed and the individual is instructed to look for the button. The leader encourages peer assistance or prompts systematic looking if the member seems to be having difficulty locating the button. One method is to walk the member around the group asking him or her to stop at each member and look from the head to the feet, both front and back.

PARTICIPATION
PROCEDURE: The first member is chosen through the BLIND SELECTION METHOD. Then, the member who finds the button becomes the next one to hide it until all members have had a turn.

TITLE: **"Which Hand?"**

SOCIALIZATION
GOAL AREA: Interpersonal Distance/Learning to be Close to Others

MATERIALS: Bag of small wrapped snacks or candy

GAME PROCEDURE: A group member conceals a single packet/piece in one hand and makes fists with both hands. He/she then walks around the inside of the circle and stops before another group member. The second member then tries to guess which hand has the packet/piece. If this member is wrong then the target group member continues around the circle and stops before another member. If the member is correct, then he/she gets the item and selects a new item and begins the game again.

PARTICIPATION
PROCEDURE: The first member is chosen through the BLIND SELECTION METHOD. Then, the member who chose correctly continues the game until all group members have had at least one turn.

TITLE: **"Working Together to Beat the Clock"**

SOCIALIZATION
GOAL AREA: Interpersonal Distance/Learning to be Close to Others

MATERIALS: Kitchen timer, ring-toss set-up, donut-shaped posterboard cut-outs

GAME PROCEDURE: A donut-shaped cut-out is passed out to each group member. The group is told that the ring-toss stand will be passed around and everyone must get their cut-out on the stand and pass it to the next person.

Group members are also told that a kitchen timer will be set. If all group members get their cut-out on the stand before the timer rings then the group gets special recognition.

PARTICIPATION
PROCEDURE: Everyone in the group has a chance to participate at the same time.

SUGGESTIONS: This game will probably take a number of practice sessions so the leader should allow time for several rounds, before setting the timer. Depending on the number of group members the timer may be adjusted from 30 + seconds.

SELF–AWARENESS
(LEARNING ABOUT MYSELF)

"Are You Happy or Are You Mad?"
"Feelings About Our Group"
"Finish the Sentence"
"Here's How I'm Feeling Today"
"Signal If You Know" I
"I Feel Really Good About . . . "
"My Favorite Things"
"Name Warm-Up"
"The Feeling Meter"
"Things We Like To Do Together"
"Do You Agree?" I
"Remember When . . . "
"Happy, Sad, or Mad"
"I Would Feel Better If . . . "
"I Blew It"
"Guess What I'm Doing"
"I Like It When . . . "
"Telling About Myself"
"Paycheck Goes Up, Paycheck Goes Down"
"Paying Attention To My Work"
"What I Really Like About My Job"
"Been There, Done That"
"Like It Or Not"
"What's Missing?"
"It's OK By Me" or, "I Want To Make A Change"

TITLE: **"Are You Happy or Are You Mad?"**

SOCIALIZATION
GOAL AREA: Self-awareness/Learning About Myself

MATERIALS: One 4″ × 6″ index card with a smile face drawn on it for each group member; one 4″ × 6″ index card with a frown face drawn on it for each group member.

GAME PROCEDURE: Members are each given two cards: one with a smile face on it and another with a frown face. Group members are told that they will be given a situation; each member must hold up the card that indicates their feeling. The situations provided by the group leader should be concrete. Some suggestions follow:

1. When I get to go shopping I feel ___.
2. When someone steals something of mine I feel ___.
3. When I get a letter in the mail I feel ___.
4. When I get a telephone call I feel ___.
5. When someone hits me I feel ___.
6. When someone helps me clean my room I feel ___.
7. When I make a new friend I feel ___.
8. When someone asks me to go out for a walk I feel ___.
9. When I get my paycheck at work I feel ___.
10. When my supervisor tells me I'm doing a good job I feel ___.

PARTICIPATION
PROCEDURE: Everyone in the group has a chance to participate at the same time.

SUGGESTIONS: The leader may want to do about ten rounds. Concrete situations can be changed to fit in with group member's interests and preferences.

TITLE: **"Feelings About Our Group"**

SOCIALIZATION
GOAL AREA: Self-awareness/Learning About Myself

MATERIALS: A "feeling meter" is made from construction paper with a pointer in the center. The meter is divided into three sections, pictorialized as happy, mad, and sad.

GAME PROCEDURE: This game is used during the termination phase of the group. A group member is presented with a structured "feeling" question and the person indicates his/her response on the "feeling meter." A member who wants to explain, discuss or elaborate on his/her feelings should have an opportunity to do so. Structured questions that leaders can use include the following:

"Do you feel happy, sad or mad . . ."

1. about being in our group?"
2. about this Game?"
3. about not having group anymore?"
4. if our group could go on?"
5. when you think of our group?"
6. about being in another group?"
7. about bringing a friend to visit our group?"

PARTICIPATION
PROCEDURE: The BLIND SELECTION METHOD is used until all members have had a turn.

TITLE: **"Finish the Sentence"**

SOCIALIZATION
GOAL AREA: Self-awareness/Learning About Myself

MATERIALS: No special materials are required

GAME PROCEDURE: The leader has a list of unfinished sentences. The leader explains to the group that he/she is going to present an unfinished sentence to a group member who is then supposed to finish it. The leader then moves quickly around the group giving each member a chance to finish a different sentence.

Examples of unfinished sentences follow:

1. On my hamburger I like . . .
2. For dessert I like . . .
3. My favorite TV show is . . .
4. My chore is . . .
5. When I need help with a problem I can go to . . .
6. For a snack I like to eat/drink . . .
7. My favorite color is . . .
8. When I have free time I like to . . .
9. For my birthday I like to . . .
10. My special wish is to . . .

PARTICIPATION
PROCEDURE: The LEADER SELECTION METHOD is used by moving around the group giving each member a turn.

TITLE: **"Here's How I'm Feeling Today"**

SOCIALIZATION
GOAL AREA: Self-awareness/Learning About Myself

MATERIALS: 3 cards depicting happy, mad, and sad faces

GAME PROCEDURE: A member draws one of the cards from the set and is instructed to act out the feeling without telling the group what it is. The leader asks the members to raise their hands if they can identify the feeling. The member identifying the feeling becomes the next participant.

PARTICIPATION
PROCEDURE: The LEADER SELECTION METHOD is used until all members have had a turn.

SUGGESTIONS: The leader may introduce the cards by passing them around the group to get members to identify the feelings represented by the cards. The leaders may also model each feeling prior to playing the game.

TITLE: **"Signal If You Know" I**

SOCIALIZATION
GOAL AREA: Self-awareness/Learning About Myself

MATERIALS: Signaling devices

GAME PROCEDURE: The leader distributes signaling devices to group members and demonstrates noise they make. Members are told that the leader will ask a question and if they have an answer they can signal with their noisemaker. All who signal will take turns answering.

Possible questions include:

1. What is your favorite thing to eat?
2. Who is your best friend?
3. What is your favorite activity?
4. What is your favorite TV show?
5. Where is your favorite place to go?
6. What is your favorite color?
7. What do you do for exercise?
8. Where do you like to shop?

PARTICIPATION
PROCEDURE: The LEADER SELECTION METHOD is used.

SUGGESTIONS: Questions can be added to fit in with the group member's interests, preferences and activities.

TITLE: **"I Feel Really Good About . . . "**

SOCIALIZATION
GOAL AREA: Self-awareness/Learning About Myself

MATERIALS: No special materials are required

GAME PROCEDURE: A group member is seated in the center of the circle. The leader presents him/her with a situation to which he/she must state whether he/she would feel good or bad about the specific situation. After the chosen member responds, group members then have an opportunity to express their feelings about the specific situation. This can be done through a group vote, e.g., leader asks "Who else feels bad about his situation?" The group member can be helped to count the number of group members who feel the same.

Suggested situations are:

"Do you feel good or bad when . . .

You are wearing your favorite outfit."
You get to go on a trip."
You get in a fight with your best friend."
Your supervisor tells you that you did a good job."
Your clothes don't fit."
Your friend invites you over for dinner."
Someone teases you."
You lose your paycheck."
You get to go to a baseball game."
You lose your wallet (or purse)."
You help your friend."
You have enough money to buy new clothes."
You oversleep and you are late for work."
You take a friend to a movie."
You go to a party."
Your friend is sick."

PARTICIPATION
PROCEDURE: The BLIND SELECTION METHOD is used.

SUGGESTIONS: The leader may want to introduce the concept of "feeling good" or "feeling bad" about oneself by suggesting that there are things that can make us feel good about ourselves.

Some of these things are:

1. helping others
2. sharing with others
3. looking clean and neat, etc.

Also, leader suggests that there are things that can make us feel bad such as:

1. arguing with friends
2. not being able to go places we want
3. not having enough money.

TITLE:	**"My Favorite Things"**
SOCIALIZATION GOAL AREA:	Self-awareness/Learning About Myself
MATERIALS:	Timer
GAME PROCEDURE:	Members are presented with a concrete category, e.g., food, and are asked to come up with something that they like within that category. The leader sets the timer and moves around the circle asking each group member to say something different within the assigned category. When the timer signals then the leader changes to a new category.

Examples of categories are:

1. Food
2. Friends
3. Favorite thing to do during spare time
4. Special wish
5. Season of the year
6. TV show
7. Favorite chair
8. Favorite place to visit
9. Snack

PARTICIPATION
PROCEDURE: The LEADER SELECTION METHOD is used by moving around the group in order, giving each member a turn.

SUGGESTIONS: Categories can be changed to fit in with group member's interests and preferences.

TITLE: "Name Warm-Up"

SOCIALIZATION
GOAL AREA: Self-awareness/Learning About Myself

MATERIALS: Standard set of photographs

GAME PROCEDURE: Each member selects his/her picture from the set and shows it to other group members. He/she is instructed to introduce himself/herself, i.e., "My name is _____" and tell about something he/she likes to do, knows how to do, or wants to learn.

PARTICIPATION
PROCEDURE: The BLIND SELECTION METHOD is used.

TITLE: "The Feeling Meter"

SOCIALIZATION
GOAL AREA: Self-awareness/Learning About Myself

MATERIALS: A feeling meter is from construction paper, with a pointer in the center. The meter is divided into three sections, pictorialized as happy, mad, and sad.

GAME PROCEDURE: The member draws a situation from a container, the "Feeling Box" and then is instructed to go to the "Feeling Meter" and point the arrow to the feeling that matches the situation.

Suggestions for situations are:

1. a teacher tells you that you did good on a test.

2. your friend calls you to talk.

3. your neighbor's dog barks and keeps you up all night.

4. your mother brings you a gift.

5. your cat dies.

6. your roommate borrows your shampoo and doesn't return it.

7. you see your girlfriend/boyfriend kissing another person.

8. you finish a puzzle that you've been working on for a long time.

9. your work friend is absent.

10. your friend calls many times each day.

11. you get a special award.

12. someone thanks you for helping them.

PARTICIPATION
PROCEDURE: The BLIND SELECTION METHOD is used until all members have had a turn.

SUGGESTIONS: For work adjustment, the following may be used:

1. My work area.

2. My supervisor.

3. My co-workers (the people I work with).

4. The building/place where I work.

5. My paycheck.

6. My job.

7. My rules at work.

8. My transportation.

TITLE: **"Things We Like To Do Together"**

SOCIALIZATION
GOAL AREA: Self-awareness/Learning About Myself

MATERIALS: Pictures of activities members could do in a group, i.e., eat, swim, picnic, take walks, dance, go to movies, etc.

GAME PROCEDURE: Leader asks members to verbalize what they do in this group; i.e. play games. Leader asks members to think about other activities the group could do together. Each member is asked to select from the activity box one of the activity pictures. Members are asked to vote whether they would like to do each activity.

PARTICIPATION
PROCEDURE: The BLIND SELECTION METHOD is used.

TITLE: **"Do You Agree?" I**

SOCIALIZATION
GOAL AREA: Self-awareness/Learning About Myself

MATERIALS: No special materials are required

GAME PROCEDURE: Members are verbally presented with a concrete activity, food or situation and they must decide whether they like it or not. If the member likes or enjoys doing the activity then he/she signals by standing, raising hands, nodding after the leader's cue.

The leader starts the game by saying:

"We are going to say some things that you all may like or may not like to do. If you like to do the things we say then you signal."

Some examples:

The leader's cue will be "Signal if you like...."

1. to eat spinach."
2. to go swimming."
3. to be teased."
4. to eat pizza."
5. to sleep late on Saturdays."
6. to go to have lunch with a friend."
7. to go to bed early."
8. to get into fights."

9. to have a good friend."
10. to be yelled at."
11. to take a walk with someone."
12. to share a secret with a friend."
13. to go on a date."

PARTICIPATION
PROCEDURE: Everyone has a chance to participate at the same time.

TITLE: **"Remember When . . ."**

SOCIALIZATION
GOAL AREA: Self-awareness/Learning About Myself

MATERIALS: 3″ × 5″ index cards depicting various activities/events

GAME PROCEDURE: Members take turns drawing an activity card. The leader assists members in sharing positive experiences similar to that pictured in the card. Each member is then asked to identify others in the group who also participated in the activity. Members are asked to raise their hands or signal to indicate that they would like to again participate in the activity in the future. Possible activities could include various jobs inside and outside of the home, shopping, movies, bowling, taking walks, cooking, exercising, hobbies, special parties, dining out, etc.

PARTICIPATION
PROCEDURE: The LEADER SELECTION METHOD is used.

SUGGESTIONS: Photographs, pictures from magazines and drawings may be used to make the game materials. Group members could assist with the process.

TITLE: "Happy, Sad or Mad"

SOCIALIZATION
GOAL AREA: Self-awareness/Learning About Myself

MATERIALS: None

GAME PROCEDURE: The leader demonstrates nonverbally the three basic feeling states of happy, sad and mad. Group members are encouraged to identify each feeling and then take turns demonstrating their own interpretation of one of the feeling states. The remaining members guess the feeling state being demonstrated.

PARTICIPATION
PROCEDURE: The BLIND or LEADER SELECTION METHOD is used until all members have had a turn.

TITLE: "I Would Feel Better If . . ."

SOCIALIZATION
GOAL AREA: Self-awareness/Learning About Myself

MATERIALS: 3″ × 5″ index cards

GAME PROCEDURE: The leader introduces the game by telling members that each will be given the chance to think about ways to change or make their situation or relationships work better. Members will then take turns responding to index cards which depict various aspects of their relationship or living arrangements by responding "no change" or one change they would make. Members will then discuss their feelings about the proposed changes.

Sample categories/aspects to consider could include:

1. The ways we talk to each other.
2. The things we do together for fun.
3. The ways we help each other.

4. The ways we work out problems.

5. The way we listen to each other.

6. The way we tell each other how we feel.

PARTICIPATION
PROCEDURE: The LEADER SELECTION METHOD is used.

TITLE: **"I Blew it"**

SOCIALIZATION
GOAL AREA: Self-awareness/Learning About Myself

MATERIALS: None

GAME PROCEDURE: Group members take turns sharing one situation in which he/she made a mistake. The leader encourages group identification and sharing related to similar experiences, related feelings and learning resulting from such experiences.

PARTICIPATION
PROCEDURE: The BLIND or LEADER SELECTION METHOD is used.

TITLE: **"Guess What I'm Doing . . . "**

SOCIALIZATION
GOAL AREA: Self-awareness/Learning About Myself

MATERIALS: None

GAME PROCEDURE: Members are instructed to physically demonstrate or "show without talking" a special activity that they enjoy. Other members try to guess the activity. If members have difficulty, they may ask questions. Once the activity is identified, the leader asks for members to raise their hands or signal if they also enjoy that activity.

Sample activities may include; household chores, recreational or social activities (i.e.

bowling, dancing, shopping). If individuals experience physical limitations that prevent effective demonstration, other group members could be selected to assist.

PARTICIPATION
PROCEDURE: The BLIND or LEADER SELECTION METHOD is used.

TITLE: "I Like It When ..."

SOCIALIZATION
GOAL AREA: Self-awareness/Learning About Myself

MATERIALS: None

GAME PROCEDURE: The leader begins by giving examples of responses to "I like it when ...." Members take turns responding to the same sentence stem. After each response, the leader can encourage members to agree or disagree or discuss the statements.

This game may be used for different relationship/friendship issues by filling in the blank with the specific descriptor (i.e., co-worker; instructor; supervisor; roommate; parent; support staff).

PARTICIPATION
PROCEDURE: The BLIND or LEADER SELECTION METHOD is used.

TITLE: "Telling About Myself"

SOCIALIZATION
GOAL AREA: Self-awareness/Learning About Myself

MATERIALS: Full length mirror, camera

GAME PROCEDURE: The group leader takes turns standing by each group member with the mirror. The leader asks each member to tell what he/she looks like. Since this is hard for some people, specific questions could be asked such as:

What color is your hair?
Is your hair short or long?
What color are your eyes?
Do you wear glasses?
What is your hairstyle?

Questions can then be directed to other group members such as "Do you notice anything else about . . . ? After each person's turn, the group leader takes a picture of that person.

PARTICIPATION
PROCEDURE: The BLIND SELECTION METHOD is used.

SUGGESTION: The leader may want to collect or retain the photographs for use throughout the group program.

TITLE: **"Paycheck Goes Up, Paycheck Goes Down"**

SOCIALIZATION
GOAL AREA: Self-awareness/Learning About Myself (work)

MATERIALS: 3″ × 5″ Index Cards

GAME PROCEDURE: Leader lists the following scenarios on individual index cards. Members take turns drawing a card and responding to the scenario with "paycheck goes up" or "paycheck goes down" depending on the probable outcome. Leader then asks other members to raise their hands, (signal) if they agree or don't agree. Members take turns until all cards are used.

Sample scenarios:

1. You have your head down on work table.
2. You are sitting at table working.
3. You are sitting at table talking to others.
4. You ask supervisor for materials.
5. You repeatedly ask to go to the bathroom.

6. You put work down and sit doing nothing.
7. You ask the boss to teach you a new job.
8. You say you don't want to work.
9. You keep working until the boss tells you to stop.
10. You walk around the work area.

PARTICIPATION
PROCEDURE: BLIND SELECTION METHOD or LEADER SELECTION METHOD may be used.

TITLE: **"Paying Attention to My Work"**

SOCIALIZATION
GOAL AREA: Self-awareness/Learning About Myself (work)

MATERIALS: 3″ × 5″ index cards with one problem scenario per card

GAME PROCEDURE: Member will take turns responding to the following scenarios presented by the leader with "This would make it hard for me to pay attention" or "This wouldn't bother me."

Sample scenarios include:

1. I had a fight with my roommate before work.
2. I have a headache.
3. I had a seizure this morning.
4. I am going shopping after work.
5. My boyfriend/girlfriend broke up with me last night.
6. My mother went in the hospital this morning.
7. My good friend died.
8. I'd like to date someone at work.
9. My co-worker talks a lot.
10. My co-worker plays his radio.
11. The phone rings a lot in my area.
12. My work area is too cold/hot.

PARTICIPATION
PROCEDURE: Everyone has a chance to participate at the same time.

TITLE: **"What I Really Like About My Job"**

SOCIALIZATION
GOAL AREA: Self-awareness/Learning About Myself (work)

MATERIALS: None

GAME PROCEDURE: Members take turns sharing one aspect of their job that they like. The leader will ask other members to raise their hand or signal if they agree or feel the same way.

PARTICIPATION
PROCEDURE: BLIND or LEADER SELECTION METHODS may be used.

SUGGESTIONS: For members who have difficulty expressing themselves verbally, the leader can use statements that require only "yes" or "no" responses. For example, putting things in bags or boxes, wiping tables, sweeping the floor, emptying trash, cleaning bathrooms, heat sealing, making salads, etc.

TITLE: **"Been There, Done That"**

SOCIALIZATION
GOAL AREA: Self-awareness/Learning About Myself

MATERIALS: Index cards with the words "Been There, Done That" for each member

GAME PROCEDURE: The leader tells group members that he/she is going to say the name of an activity and they are to respond by holding up their cards, if they have previously participated in the activity. If members have not participated in the activity the card is to remain in their laps.

The leader then asks members whose cards are in their laps, if they would like to participate in the activity and proceeds to make a list of new activities that members would like to experience.

PARTICIPATION
PROCEDURE: Everyone has a chance to participate at the same time.

SUGGESTIONS: Leaders may expand the activity by including magazine pictures of activities that can be used to make a group collage. Activity lists may also be given to members to be placed in their folders or taken home.

Sample activities include:

1. outdoor concert
2. trip to another city or state
3. phone call to friend
4. plan visit to friend's house
5. boating
6. theater/plays
7. make a video
8. tape music
9. plant a garden
10. hiking/nature walks
11. church/synagogue activities
12. special festivals/events
13. fishing
14. galleries/museums
15. video/computer games and activities
16. volunteer activities
17. movies
18. shopping
19. order pizza
20. camp

TITLE: **"Like It Or Not"**

SOCIALIZATION
GOAL AREA: Self-awareness/Learning About Myself

MATERIALS: 3″ × 5″ index cards for each member with the words "Like it" or a smiling face

GAME PROCEDURE: The group leader tells members that they are going to hear about things that they may like or not. In response to each item, members are asked to raise their cards if they "like it" or keep them in their laps if they don't. The leader and members, if possible, take turns reading the items. Members are encouraged to identify others in the group who feel like they do and those who do not in a turn-taking format. The game ends when all items have been presented.

PARTICIPATION
PROCEDURE: Group members participate at the same time.

SUGGESTIONS: Items can include foods, clothing types, activities, weather conditions and situations specific to the program environment or theme (i.e., recess, gym, or homework in school settings and learning new jobs, getting a raise, and receiving praise in a work setting). Members can also be encouraged to come up with their own items for the group.

TITLE: **"What's Missing?"**

SOCIALIZATION
GOAL AREA: Self-awareness/Learning About Myself

MATERIALS: Tray and a number of small objects

GAME PROCEDURE: The leader arranges four or five items on a tray and shows them to all members. One member is selected to remove one of the objects while a second member turns away or is blindfolded. The second member must then try to remember what is missing. Group members are encouraged to give hints or provide assistance, if necessary. The game continues until everyone has had a turn.

PARTICIPATION
PROCEDURE: The BLIND or LEADER SELECTION METHOD is used.

SUGGESTIONS: Objects may be changed after several turns to keep the game challenging.

TITLE: "It's OK By Me or, I Want To Make A Change"

SOCIALIZATION
GOAL AREA: Self-awareness/Learning About Myself

MATERIALS: 3″ × 5″ index cards

GAME PROCEDURE: Members take turns responding to index cards that depict different aspects of their relationship by responding "It's OK" or "I want to make a change." Members wanting to make a change are asked to suggest one type of change that would make things better. Other members are encouraged to respond and/or provide other suggestions for making things better.

Sample scenarios are:

1. The way we talk to each other.
2. The way we treat each other.
3. The way we share with each other.
4. The way we work out problems together.
5. The way we do fun things together.
6. The way we work together.
7. The way _____

PARTICIPATION
PROCEDURE: BLIND or LEADER SELECTION METHOD is used.

SOCIAL AWARENESS (LEARNING ABOUT OTHERS)

"Back-to-Back"
"Can You Pretend?"
"Clothing Color Match"
"Find the Owner"
"Find Your Friend"
"Find the Person"
"Signal If You Know" II
"I Know Something About You"
"If I Were You"
"Name Draw"
"Name Game" I
"Name Game" II
"Pick a Friend"
"Seeing the Best"
"The Blindfold Game"
"TV Star"
"We Had a Great Group!"
"We Have A Lot in Common"
"Whisper"
"Who Am I Talking About?"
"Who Is This Person?"
"Who's Missing?"
"Guess Who?" II
"I Know Something Good About . . . "
"Guess My Job"
"Birthday Box"
"Do You Agree?" II
"Good For You"

TITLE: **"Back-To-Back"**

SOCIALIZATION
GOAL AREA: Social Awareness/Learning About Others

MATERIALS: No special materials are required

GAME PROCEDURE: Two members sit back-to-back in the center of the group. The first member selected tells the group something that his/her partner is wearing. If he/she is correct the partner signals, (claps and raises hands). The participant must then tell some thing different that the partner is wearing in order to complete the turn. Roles are then reversed.

PARTICIPATION
PROCEDURE: The BLIND SELECTION METHOD is used to select two members at a time until all members have had a turn.

TITLE: **"Can You Pretend?"**

SOCIALIZATION
GOAL AREA: Social Awareness/Learning About Others

MATERIALS: No special materials are required

GAME PROCEDURE: A group member is selected to draw a name of another group member from a box. The leader tells the name of this group member to the selected member and tells him/her to make believe he/she is this person. The goal is to demonstrate something special about the person. The group then tries to guess who is being imitated by the selected member.

PARTICIPATION
PROCEDURE: The first member is selected through the BLIND SELECTION METHOD. Once the group member who is being imitated is identified he/she gets the next turn until all members have had a turn.

SUGGESTIONS: The leader may suggest that members act out a special interest, skill, activity.

TITLE: **"Clothing Color Match"**

SOCIALIZATION
GOAL AREA: Social Awareness/Learning About Others

MATERIALS: Ten index cards; each card has one of the following colors on it: black, blue, red, brown, yellow, green, orange, pink, gold, white. (Note: colors can be put on cards with crayons)

GAME PROCEDURE: Index cards are placed in a box. A group member selects a card from the box and identifies the color. The member then walks around group and attempts to find another member who is wearing some piece of clothing that contains the chosen color.

PARTICIPATION
PROCEDURE: The BLIND SELECTION METHOD is used to select the initial person. Thereafter, the person who is identified as wearing the selected color gets the opportunity to draw a card from the box. This continues until all group members have had a turn.

SUGGESTION: The leader may want to bring a box of crayons and a small supply of index cards into the group. The leader should scan the group to see what colors are being worn. The leader can then make up some additional cards if necessary. By scanning beforehand, the leader will insure that each member will be chosen.

TITLE: **"Find the Owner"**

SOCIALIZATION
GOAL AREA: Social Awareness/Knowing About Others

MATERIALS: Box containing objects belonging to group members, e.g., watch, necklace, ring, cup, key, barrette, book, etc., blindfold

GAME PROCEDURE: Members are asked to place one of their personal possessions in the group box. A member is then asked to choose an item from the box without looking. The member must return the object to its proper owner.

PARTICIPATION
PROCEDURE: The BLIND SELECTION METHOD is used until all members have had a turn.

TITLE: "Find Your Friend"

SOCIALIZATION
GOAL AREA: Social Awareness/Knowing About Others

MATERIALS: Blindfold, standard pictures (see p. 51)

GAME PROCEDURE: One member is blindfolded. Another member selects a picture from all pictures with faces down and leads the blindfolded member around the circle to locate this member. The pair is instructed to stop at each member who in turn is to say "Hi." The leading member then inquires "Is this Sue?" and continues around the group until the individual is identified.

PARTICIPATION
PROCEDURE: The BLIND SELECTION METHOD is used.

TITLE: "Find The Person"

SOCIALIZATION
GOAL AREA: Social-awareness/Learning About Others

MATERIALS: Twenty index cards are needed. These cards are divided up into two piles of ten cards each. One pile of cards represent personal objects.

A picture is sketched on each card with pencil or crayon. These pictures can include: (1) glasses; (2) pocketbook; (3) dress; (4) slacks; (5) earrings; (6) ring/jewelry; (7) socks; (8) tennis shoes; (9) hat; and (10) shorts. Another set of cards, personal characteristic, can contain pictures of the following: (1) a face with freckles; (2) a person with short hair; (3) a person with long hair; (4) a face with a smile; (5) a person wearing braided hair; (6) a short person standing next to a tall person; (7) a person with blonde hair; (8) a person with brown hair; (9) a skinny person, and (10) a person with straight hair

GAME PROCEDURE: The set of "personal object" cards are placed in a box. A group member selects a card from the box, and identifies the object. The member then walks around the group and locates another member who has the selected object. After the "personal object" cards are used, then the "personal characteristic" cards are placed in the box.

PARTICIPATION
PROCEDURES: The BLIND SELECTION METHOD is used to select the initial person. Thereafter the person who is identified as having the selected object or characteristic gets the opportunity to draw a card from the box.

SUGGESTIONS: This game requires that the leader know group members fairly well. The personal objects and characteristics listed above were designed for a group whose membership were women. Other leaders may feel that these are not appropriate for a particular group, so other objects and characteristics can be developed. For instance, a group of men, the following could be used: (1) a person with a mustache; (2) a person with a beard; (3) a person smoking a pipe. The important point is that the leader should get members to observe the personal characteristics of other people.

TITLE:	**"Signal If You Know" II**
SOCIALIZATION GOAL AREA:	Social Awareness/Learning About Others
MATERIALS:	Signaling Device
GAME PROCEDURE:	The leader starts off game by signaling and saying, "I know something about (Sally)! She (likes to go to the store), (doesn't like coffee), (wants to go to the zoo), (has a new sweater), (etc.). The leader then opens up the game to the group by saying, "If anyone else can tell us something about (Sally) you can sound the signal and tell us."
PARTICIPATION PROCEDURE:	The LEADER or BLIND SELECTION METHOD is used until each group member has had a turn.
SUGGESTION:	The leader may want to remind members to share positive or nice comments.

TITLE:	**"I Know Something About You"**
SOCIALIZATION GOAL AREA:	Social Awareness/Learning About Others
MATERIALS:	Blindfold
GAME PROCEDURE:	Two members are seated in the center of the circle and given 30 seconds to look at each other. Following the time limit, they are blindfolded one at a time and asked questions about each other. Each right answer is rewarded with applause. Sample questions are:

What color is your partners hair?
Does he/she have glasses on?
Does he/she have a dress or pants on?
Does he/she have shoes on?
Does he/she have on the color red?
What style is her/his hair?

PARTICIPATION
PROCEDURE: The BLIND SELECTION METHOD is used picking two members at a time.

TITLE: "If I Were You"

SOCIALIZATION
GOAL AREA: Social Awareness/Learning About Others

MATERIALS: No special materials required

GAME PROCEDURE: Two members are selected. The leader asks the first member to tell or show the group something that the other member does. Each member must contribute something different with prompting from the group permissible. To decrease the difficulty level of the game it is suggested that the facilitators provide categories of activities, i.e., work/job, recreation, hobbies.

PARTICIPATION
PROCEDURE: The BLIND SELECTION METHOD is recommended with each member in turn selecting the next participant.

TITLE: "Name Game" I

SOCIALIZATION
GOAL AREA: Social Awareness/Learning About Others

MATERIALS: Bean bag or other soft ball

GAME PROCEDURE: Each member is instructed to call out the name of someone in the group before tossing the object to them. The game proceeds with members catching the object and then throwing it to another member.

PARTICIPATION
PROCEDURE: Starting member is selected by BLIND SELECTION METHOD.

TITLE: **"Name Game" II**

SOCIALIZATION
GOAL AREA: Social Awareness/Learning About Others

MATERIALS: Bean bag or other soft ball; timer, standard pictures

GAME PROCEDURE: One member is selected as a name caller and calls members' names one at a time by pulling from pictures. As he/she calls the name, the person with the bag/ball throws it to the named individual. The caller continues until the timer rings. The timer should be set for from 3–5 minutes to permit each member to be a caller.

PARTICIPATION
PROCEDURE: The BLIND SELECTION METHOD is used.

TITLE: **"Pick A Friend"**

SOCIALIZATION
GOAL AREA: Social Awareness/Learning About Others

MATERIALS: No special materials are required

GAME PROCEDURE: A group member is selected and seated in the center of the circle. The selected member is instructed to look around the group at each member's clothing. He/she is told to select a person, but not say the name. The selected member gives a clue about the person by saying something about the color of his/her clothing. For example, the seated member says: "I am thinking of someone wearing blue shoes." Everyone tries to identify the person.

When correctly identified, the person comes up and shakes the member's hand and then takes the center seat.

PARTICIPATION
PROCEDURE: The BLIND SELECTION METHOD is used to select one group member at a time.

SUGGESTIONS: The center member could be given something (i.e. small wrapped item) to share with the selected member.

TITLE: **"Seeing The Best"**

SOCIALIZATION
GOAL AREA: Social Awareness/Learning About Others

MATERIALS: Sunglasses or fun glasses

GAME PROCEDURE: The leader shows the group the sunglasses and says, "When we wear these we see only good things about others." Two members sit in the middle of the group facing each other. One member puts on the "glasses" and is asked to think of something to say to make his/her partner happy, e.g., say something friendly. Then the roles are reversed and the partner must put on the "glasses."

PARTICIPATION
PROCEDURE: The BLIND SELECTION METHOD is used to select two members at a time until all have had a turn.

SUGGESTIONS: For members having difficulty with this task, other group members may be asked to assist.

TITLE: **"The Blindfold Game"**

SOCIALIZATION
GOAL AREA: Social Awareness/Learning About Others

MATERIALS: Blindfold

GAME PROCEDURE: One group member is seated before the group and is blindfolded. Another member is selected to sit beside the blindfolded person. This person gives an auditory cue by saying "Hi." The blindfolded person is then given a chance to guess the identity of the person. If necessary, repeated or expanded verbalizations may be given.

PARTICIPATION
PROCEDURE: The blindfolded member is selected through the BLIND SELECTION METHOD. The other member is selected by the LEADER SELECTION METHOD.

TITLE: "TV Star"

SOCIALIZATION
GOAL AREA: Social Awareness/Learning About Others

MATERIALS: Standard photographs of each group member, a television screen drawn on a cardboard with slits so that a photograph can be placed in the screen

GAME PROCEDURE: A group member's photograph is selected from a box of photos. The person is identified by another group member and it is announced that this is "The (Sally Wilson) television show." The leader then places the photograph in the television screen. The "TV Star" is asked to come before group. The group is then asked, "What do you like about this person?" When group members contribute positive comments then the "TV Star" thanks the contributor and shakes his/her hand.

PARTICIPATION
PROCEDURE: The BLIND SELECTION METHOD is used to select the "TV Star."

SUGGESTIONS: This game depends on the leader playing up the idea that the group members will be "TV Stars." It is beneficial if the leader plays up a group member having his/her own television show and the leader should work at making the selected person the center of attention.

TITLE: **"We Had a Great Group"**

SOCIALIZATION
GOAL AREA: Social Awareness/Learning About Others

MATERIALS: Group pictures of all members

GAME PROCEDURE: The leader holds up the group picture and presents a riddle about each member, telling members for example, "This great group member likes (to sing)," etc. The member who guesses the identity takes a group picture from the leader and presents it to the member. Members are encouraged to clap for each person "who was a really great group member." The procedure continues until all have received a group picture.

PARTICIPATION
PROCEDURE: LEADER SELECTION METHOD is used.

TITLE: **"We Have A Lot In Common"**

SOCIALIZATION
GOAL AREA: Social Awareness/Learning About Others

MATERIALS: No special materials are required

GAME PROCEDURE: The leader explains to group members that there are many ways that we are all alike and many ways that we are different. Two stations or areas are set up on opposite sides of the members' circle. The leader then tells the members that "We are going to find out how we are alike and how we are different." The leader resents members with forced-choice characteristics. If the members have the characteristic, they are instructed to go to one of the stations. If not, they go to the other. The leader then draws attention to the fact that, "This is a way in which some of us are different," or "This is a way in which we are all alike."

The following categories/characteristics could be used in this game:

1. Gender
2. Hair color/Hair style
3. Height—tall or short
4. Activity interests
5. Wears glasses or doesn't wear glasses/jewelry
6. Living arrangements
7. Likes specific types of food
8. Favorite color

PARTICIPATION
PROCEDURE: All group members participate simultaneously.

SUGGESTIONS: Questions can be added to fit in with the group member's interests, preferences and activities.

TITLE: "Whisper"

SOCIALIZATION
GOAL AREA: Social Awareness/Learning About Others

MATERIALS: Blindfold

GAME PROCEDURE: A group member is blindfolded and placed in the middle of the group. Another member is selected to go up to the blindfolded member and whisper something in his/her ear. The "whispering" member then returns to his/her seat. The blindfold is removed and the member is asked to point to the one who he/she thinks whispered to him/her. If the member is correct, the game proceeds until all members have had a turn. If the member is wrong, the original blindfold process is repeated.

PARTICIPATION
PROCEDURE: The BLIND SELECTION METHOD is used.

SUGGESTIONS: To encourage involvement, the group may be encouraged to say "yes" or "no" after the blindfolded member makes his/her choice.

TITLE: **"Who Am I Talking About?"**

SOCIALIZATION
GOAL AREA: Social Awareness/Learning About Others

MATERIALS: Full length photo of each member

GAME PROCEDURE: A group member is seated in the center of the group and asked to select one photo from the group of photos. The member is instructed to look at the photo so that he/she can answer some questions about the person pictured.

The following questions may be used:

1. Is this person a man or woman?
2. Is this person tall or short?
3. Does this person have long or short hair?
4. Does this person wear glasses?
5. Does this person have a beard or mustache (if applicable)?
6. Does this person have curly or straight hair?

After each question, the leader asks the rest of the group to guess the identity of the person described; and to raise their hands if they know. Whoever correctly guesses goes into the center of the group for his/her turn.

PARTICIPATION
PROCEDURE: The LEADER SELECTION METHOD is used until all members have had a turn.

TITLE: **"Who Is This Person?"**

SOCIALIZATION
GOAL AREA: Social Awareness/Learning About Others

MATERIALS: Standard set of pictures

GAME PROCEDURE: The leader passes a photograph around the circle, of which the head is not visible (covered with paper). Each group member is asked to look at the photograph and try to think who the person is without telling the group. The leader then walks around the circle tapping different members and asking the group to raise their hands if the "mystery person" is being tapped. When the "mystery person" is correctly identified, he/she is asked to come into the center of the group to display his/her picture.

PARTICIPATION
PROCEDURE: The leader uses the BLIND SELECTION METHOD, drawing one picture at a time from the group of pictures placed face down. The game continues until all members have had a turn as the "mystery person."

TITLE: **"Who's Missing?"**

SOCIALIZATION
GOAL AREA: Social Awareness/Learning About Others

MATERIALS: No special materials are required

GAME PROCEDURE: Group members are instructed to close their eyes. The leader explains that he/she will tap someone on the shoulder and then lead that person away from the group. Group members are then told to open their eyes and look around the group to try to guess "who's missing."

PARTICIPATION
PROCEDURE: The LEADER SELECTION METHOD is used until all members have had a turn.

SUGGESTIONS: Leadership can rotate among those members who are interested.

TITLE: **"Guess Who?" II**

SOCIALIZATION
  GOAL AREA: Social Awareness/Learning About Others

MATERIALS: Tape recorder with taped messages or sounds (i.e., laughter, singing, etc.) from each group member. (each sample should be separated by approximately 5 sec. of blank tape)

GAME PROCEDURE: The leader plays a taped vocal sample to the member selected. The member is asked to guess who is talking or making the sounds. If the member has difficulty, the taped message will be replayed. Other members can then be asked to assist with identification of the member.

PARTICIPATION
  PROCEDURE: The BLIND or LEADER SELECTION METHOD may be used until each member has had a turn.

SUGGESTIONS: Group members can assist with obtaining the vocal samples of one another and other identifiable individuals in the environment (i.e., support staff, family members, friends). Leaders may want to maintain a master list of the voices in the event that members are unable to identify them.

TITLE: **"I Know Something Good About . . . "**

SOCIALIZATION
  GOAL AREA: Social Awareness/Learning About Others

MATERIALS: Streamers or other art materials to decorate a chair

GAME PROCEDURE: Group members take turns sitting in the decorated chair. This is a "special" seat and only good things can be said. The leader directs the group members to each say one good thing about the person sitting in the seat. If someone has trouble thinking of a good thing to say, the leader can give cues/hints/suggestions.

PARTICIPATION
PROCEDURE: The BLIND SELECTION METHOD is used.

SUGGESTIONS: Group members could participate in making and/or attaching decorations to the seat of honor.

TITLE: **"Guess My Job"**

SOCIALIZATION
GOAL AREA: Self-awareness/Learning About Others

MATERIALS: Job materials may be used, but are not necessary. (i.e., broom, towel, hairnet, jig, etc.)

GAME PROCEDURE: Members take turns physically demonstrating or showing others how they do their job. After each demonstration, the leader asks other group members to guess the job. If members have difficulty, they may ask questions of the person demonstrating.

PARTICIPATION
PROCEDURE: The BLIND SELECTION or LEADER SELECTION METHODS may be used.

SUGGESTIONS: The leader may want to make a list of members and their jobs for review at later sessions.

TITLE: **"Birthday Box"**

SOCIALIZATION
GOAL AREA: Social Awareness/Learning About Others

MATERIALS: Box; magazines/index cards with cut-out pictures of various objects or experiences

GAME PROCEDURE: The leader identifies the member with the birthday and asks him/her to sit in the center of the group. The leader then puts all of the cards face down in the box. Members take turns responding to the phrase "If I could, I would give you ＿＿＿＿＿ for your birth—
                                    (card)
day" while drawing a card. The member then hands the card to the birthday person. The individual responds as to how he/she feels about the gift. Other group members are then asked to signal if they agree or disagree.

PARTICIPATION
PROCEDURE: The BLIND SELECTION METHOD is used.

SUGGESTIONS: Cut-out pictures can include the following:

Pets, vacations, clothing items, jewelry, books, video, make-up, athletic equipment, funny/unusual items (i.e., Mr. Potatohead, toilet bowl, wild animal)

TITLE: **"Do You Agree?" II**

SOCIALIZATION
GOAL AREA: Social Awareness/Learning About Others

MATERIALS: None

GAME PROCEDURE: Members are verbally presented with a series of behavioral descriptions and must decide if they agree or disagree. If the member agrees then he/she signals by standing, raising hands, nodding or other means. The leader starts the game by saying:

"We are going to say some things that people do. You must decide if you think it's ok or not for a friend to do these things."

The following descriptions may be used:

1. Friend asks you to steal for them.
2. Friend asks you again and again for money, cigarettes and never pays you back.
3. Friend shares pizza with you.
4. Friend borrows $1.00 and pays you back the next week.
5. Person flirts and is *very* friendly with your boyfriend/girlfriend.
6. Friend threatens to hurt you.
7. Friend helps you when you're not feeling well.
8. Friend says bad things about you to others.
9. Friend calls to ask you to go out to eat.
10. Friend uses your things without asking.

PARTICIPATION
PROCEDURE: Everyone has a chance to participate at the same time.

TITLE: **"Good For You"**

SOCIALIZATION
GOAL AREA: Social Awareness/Learning About Others

MATERIALS: Mock award certificates (computer generated) for each group member

GAME PROCEDURE: The leader tells group members that everyone is going to receive a special certificate for special things that they do. Members take turns selecting a certificate and going to the center of the circle. Other group members are asked to share special things about the person which the leader writes on the certificate. Members take turns until all have received certificates.

PARTICIPATION
PROCEDURE: The BLIND or LEADER SELECTION METHOD is used.

PROSOCIAL
(LEARNING TO GET ALONG WITH OTHERS)

"Friendship Chain"
"Helping Each Other"
"Helping My Friend Find His/Her Stuff"
"Helping My Friend" I
"Helping My Friend" II
"I Have a Problem . . . How Can You Help?" I
"The Magic Box" I
"The Magic Box" II
"Do I Care to Share?"
"How Others Feel"
"Helping Others Feel Good"
"Friendly or Not"
"I Have a Problem . . . How Can You Help?" II
"What Am I Doing?"
"Good Times We Shared"
"What Works For Me"
"We All Win"
"Doin' The Spring Thing"

TITLE: **"Friendship Chain"**

SOCIALIZATION
GOAL AREA: Prosocial/Learning to Get Along With Others

MATERIALS: Piece of string approximately 3 feet long for each member

GAME PROCEDURE: A member stands in the middle of the circle and is asked to tell the group something he/she could do for a friend. The group is instructed to vote "OK" or "NOT." If "OK" the individual is given the first string or link of the "Friendship Chain." If "NOT" the individual is asked to try again. Another member then comes into the center of the circle and must tell the group something different that he/she would do for a friend. If correct, he/she is given his/her string and it is tied to the string of the original member.

PARTICIPATION
PROCEDURE: Turns will be by seating order until all members are linked to the "Friendship Chain."

TITLE: **"Helping Each Other"**

SOCIALIZATION
GOAL AREA: Prosocial/Learning to Get Along With Others

MATERIALS: Pairs of objects that may be used together are separated into two boxes, e.g., necklace and bracelet, comb and brush, pen and paper, toothbrush and toothpaste, soap and towel, cup and pop can, (matched clothing may be used)

GAME PROCEDURE: One member is blindfolded. Each remaining member takes turns selecting an item from one of the boxes. The blindfolded member selects an item from the match box. The blindfold is removed and the member must then locate the individual who has an item that can be used with or compliments the selected item.

PARTICIPATION
PROCEDURE: The BLIND SELECTION METHOD is used with the matching member becoming the next to be blindfolded.

TITLE: **"Helping My Friend Find His/Her Stuff"**

SOCIALIZATION
GOAL AREA: Prosocial/Learning to Get Along With Others

MATERIALS: Various small articles that may be hidden, e.g., cup, watch, book, purse (personal articles of group members may be used)

GAME PROCEDURE: One group member is escorted away from the group, preferably out of the room, but may stand with back towards group. A second group member is instructed to hide an article. The removed member is brought back to the group and instructed to find his/her missing article. The group is instructed to assist by saying "warmer" as the member approaches the hidden article, or "colder" if the member moves away from the article. After the article is located, the game proceeds until all members have had a turn.

PARTICIPATION
PROCEDURE: The BLIND SELECTION METHOD is used.

SUGGESTION: The leader may request that the searching member pause at regular intervals at which time the group is asked and prompted if necessary to indicate "warmer" or "colder."

TITLE: **"Helping My Friend" I**

SOCIALIZATION
GOAL AREA: Prosocial/Learning to Get Along With Others

MATERIALS: Assortment of items which correspond with problems presented such as umbrella, comb, hat, glove, sunglasses, hand lotion, boots, magazine, cassette tape, snack, sweater, after-have/perfume, pen

GAME PROCEDURE: Group members are told that this is a game to discover how we can help our friends. A group member comes up and sits before the group. Materials are laid out on the table. The leader then says "Our friend _____ is stuck out in the rain. Can anyone find a way to help her?" The leader then selects a member who raises his/her hand to come up and solve the problem for the target group member.

The leader continues this strategy with different members sitting before the group. Problems presented to the group can involve:

1. Your friend is cold.
2. Your friend's hair is messy.
3. Your friend's hands are dirty.
4. Your friend's eyes are bothered by the sun.
5. Your friend needs to walk in the snow.
6. Your friend is bored.
7. Your friend's skin is dry.
8. Your friend is hungry.
9. Your friend is getting ready for a special party.
10. Your friend needs to sign important papers.

PARTICIPATION
PROCEDURE: The LEADER SELECTION METHOD is used.

TITLE: "Helping My Friend" II

SOCIALIZATION
GOAL AREA: Prosocial/Learning to Get Along With Others

MATERIALS: No special materials are required.

GAME PROCEDURE: A group member is seated before the group. The leader provides a hypothetical situation: "Here's (Cindy). She can't find anything to do and she is bored. Can anyone find her something to do?" A group member is then selected to help the target member.

Hypothetical situations the leader can use include:

1. "Here's _____. He's/She's really angry. What can someone do to make him/her feel better?"
2. "Here's _____. He's/She's having a seizure. How can we help?"
3. "Here's _____. He's/She's feeling sad. What can someone do to make him/her feel better?"
4. "Here's _____. He/She has cut her finger. How can someone help him/her?"
5. "Here's _____. He/She is really cold. Who can help him/her?"
6. "Here's _____. He's/She's sick to her stomach. Who can help him/her?"
7. "Here's _____. He/She tells you that she's very thirsty. How can you help him/her?"
8. "Here's _____. He/She is lonely. How can you help him/her?"

PARTICIPATION
PROCEDURE: One group member is selected each time through the BLIND SELECTION METHOD.

TITLE: **"I Have a Problem . . . How Can You Help? I"**

SOCIALIZATION
GOAL AREA: Prosocial/Learning to Get Along With Others

MATERIALS: No special materials are required

GAME PROCEDURE: A group member is given a problem by the leader and asked "how can you help?" Other members are asked if they agree or have other suggestions.

Possible problem situations:

1. Needs to brush his/her hair but can't find a brush.
2. Can't zip a back zipper.
3. Needs a cup for coffee.
4. Hurt his/her hand and can't make the bed without help.
5. Is sick in bed and would like some water.
6. Needs to move something heavy.
7. Wants to be alone.
8. Wants to play a game.
9. Lost his/her wallet/purse.
10. Is feeling lonely.

PARTICIPATION
PROCEDURE: The LEADER SELECTION METHOD is used.

SUGGESTIONS: This game can be personalized for group members in order to promote their interpersonal problem solving.

TITLE: "The Magic Box" I

SOCIALIZATION
GOAL AREA: Prosocial/Learning to Get Along With Others

MATERIALS: Standard photographs of each group member, box with small wrapped snacks or coins

GAME PROCEDURE: Before the game is introduced, the leader tapes two candies or coins to the back of each picture. The leader explains that he/she is going to pass around a "Magic Box." A member selects a picture, identifies the person, and then shares the prize with the person.

PARTICIPATION
PROCEDURE: The BLIND SELECTION METHOD is used until all members have had a turn.

TITLE: **"The Magic Box" II**

SOCIALIZATION
GOAL AREA: Prosocial/Learning to Get Along With Others

MATERIALS: Standard photographs of each group member, attached photos or magazine pictures depicting two people participating in an activity

GAME PROCEDURE: Before the start of the session, the leader tapes one of the activities to the back of each picture. The leader explains that he/she is going to pass the "Magic Box" to one member. The member is instructed to draw a picture and then act out the activity with that individual.

PARTICIPATION
PROCEDURE: The BLIND SELECTION METHOD is used with each person drawn in turn drawing the next participant.

SUGGESTIONS: Sample activities could include:

1. Dancing
2. Talking on the phone
3. Playing Cards
4. Cooking
5. Shaking hands/greeting
6. Playing ball/tennis
7. Reading or showing pictures
8. Singing
9. Eating
10. Exercising

TITLE: **"Do I Care to Share?"**

SOCIALIZATION
GOAL AREA: Prosocial/Learning to Get Along With Others

MATERIALS: 3″ × 5″ cards with one problem scenario per card

GAME PROCEDURE: Members take turns drawing one problem card. The member, or leader, if necessary, reads the card and the member decides how to respond. Other group members are encouraged to express their ideas or suggestions.

Hypothetical problem situations the leader can use include:

1. You and a friend see a dollar on the ground.
2. You and a friend bought a pizza, there is one piece left and you both want it.
3. Your friend comes to visit and is chilly, but has no jacket.
4. You just made a pot of coffee and your friends stop over to see you.
5. You just got paid and your friend spent all of his/her money and wants you to take him/her shopping.
6. You just bought a pack of candy/cigarettes and a group of co-workers ask you to share.
7. You brought your lunch to work and your friend forgot his/hers.
8. Your friend asks to borrow your favorite watch or jewelry item.

PARTICIPATION
PROCEDURE: The BLIND SELECTION METHOD is used.

TITLE: "How Others Feel"

SOCIALIZATION
GOAL AREA: Prosocial/Learning to Get Along With Others

MATERIALS: 3″ × 5″ cards for each member depicting happy and mad faces on each side

GAME PROCEDURE: Two members at a time take turns drawing scenarios which require one member to do something for or say something to the other member. Other group members are asked to hold up their cards showing how each responding individual felt as the result of the action. Members are encouraged to share similar experiences.

SUGGESTED
SITUATIONS:

1. Loudly telling the person he/she did a very bad thing.
2. Telling the person that he/she really looks nice.
3. Teasing the person about their job (i.e. "My job is better than yours").
4. Asking the person to do something with you. (go out to eat, go to a movie, take a walk).
5. Offering to help the person change their furniture around.
6. Threatening to tell the person's boss (mother) that the person didn't do his/her job.
7. Telling the person that he/she did a good job.
8. Asking the person if they'd like a cup of coffee or pop when you get yours.
9. Walking away from a person who is trying to talk to you.
10. Giving the person a card on their birthday.
11. Making a face at the person.

PARTICIPATION
PROCEDURE: The LEADER SELECTION METHOD is used until all members have had a turn.

TITLE: **"Helping Others Feel Good"**

SOCIALIZATION
GOAL AREA: Prosocial/Learning to Get Along With Others

MATERIALS: 3″ × 5″ cards, each card to list a situation

GAME PROCEDURE: Each member draws a situation in which he/she could use help from others. Another member must think of one way to help. Other members are encouraged to think of different ways to help the individual.

Suggested situations:

1. _____ is getting ready to move to another
   (name of member drawing card)
   home.

2. _____ has returned from the store with too many packages for him/her to carry.

3. _____ is sick and can't do his/her chore.

4. _____ slipped and fell down.

5. _____ doesn't have anything to do and is bored.

6. _____ is sad that a friend has moved.

7. Someone calls on the phone for _____ but he/she is not home.

8. It is really early in the morning and _____ ran out of shampoo.

9. _____ would like to have a friend spend some time alone in your room.

10. _____ lost his/her keys in the house.

SUGGESTIONS: Present situations with both instances of an individual helping and refusing to help. Encourage the group to judge whether the behavior was helpful or not and suggest better ways of handling the situation.

TITLE: "Friendly or Not"

SOCIALIZATION
GOAL AREA: Prosocial/Learning to Get Along With Others

MATERIALS: No specific materials are needed

GAME PROCEDURE: The group leader presents various scenarios to group members and they vote "friendly" or "not." The leader is encouraged to enact scenarios when presented.

Some scenarios might be:

1. You say, "Hi!" when you pass a co-worker.
2. You give a friend a "high five" when you see him at the ballgame.
3. You raise your fist when you see your roommate at dinner.
4. You smile at a friend.
5. You slam the door in someone's face.
6. You ask a co-worker to please move out of the way.
7. You tell someone to "shut-up."
8. You ask your roommate if you can help him take out the trash.

PARTICIPATION PROCEDURE: Everyone in the group has a chance to participate at the same time.

TITLE: **"I Have A Problem . . . How Can You Help?" II**

SOCIALIZATION GOAL AREA: Prosocial (work)/Learning to Get Along With Others

MATERIALS: No special materials are required

GAME PROCEDURE: A group member is given a problem by the leader and asked "How can you help?" Other members are asked if they agree or have other suggestions.

The following problems may be used:

1. One co-worker can't reach a paper she dropped.
2. A co-worker fell down.
3. Supervisor is too busy to get materials you need.
4. The phone is ringing.
5. A co-worker lost her money in the pop machine.

6. Someone is looking for your supervisor.

7. You see smoke coming from the wastebasket.

8. A co-worker's wheelchair is blocked by some boxes.

PARTICIPATION
PROCEDURE: The LEADER SELECTION METHOD is used.

TITLE: **"What Am I Doing?"**

SOCIALIZATION
GOAL AREA: Prosocial/Learning to Get Along With Others

MATERIALS: No special materials are required

GAME PROCEDURE: A member is selected and instructed by the leader (away from the group) to go into the center of the group and "Show us a _____." Group members are then encouraged to guess what or who the member is acting like and raise their hands if they know.

Some suggested situations are:

1. person driving a car."
2. a swimmer."
3. person making a bed."
4. person mopping the floor."
5. person eating a meal."
6. person cooking a meal."
7. person drawing a picture."
8. person exercising."
9. person bowling, golfing, etc."
10. person dealing cards."

PARTICIPATION
PROCEDURE: The BLIND SELECTION METHOD is used until all members have had a turn.

SUGGESTIONS: A more advanced version may involve the selection of two members who participate in cooperative role plays. Possible role plays include throwing and catching a ball, playing cards, dancing, carrying something large, talking on the phone to each other.

TITLE:	**"Good Times We Shared"**
SOCIALIZATION GOAL AREA:	Prosocial/Learning to Get Along With Others
MATERIALS:	Index cards which depict various events/ activities
GAME PROCEDURE:	The leader tells members that this game will require them to think about things they did together in the past that they liked or enjoyed. Members take turns drawing topic cards and then share a related activity or experience that they participated in together. Activities/ events could include: Cooking projects, crafts, movies, out to eat, vacations, parties, concerts, shopping.
PARTICIPATION PROCEDURE:	The BLIND or LEADER SELECTION METHOD is used.

TITLE:	**"What Works For Me"**
SOCIALIZATION GOAL AREA:	Prosocial/Learning to Get Along With Others
MATERIALS:	Index cards listing scenarios
GAME PROCEDURE:	The leader tells members that this game will require them to think about the ways they get along with each other and what they could do to make things better between them. Members take turns drawing scenario cards and responding with "this works for me" or "this doesn't work for me." If the member responds with "this doesn't work for me," he/she is then asked to suggest a change to make things work better. Sample scenarios include:

1. The way we talk to each other.
2. The way we cooperate and share.
3. The way we help each other.
4. The way we do fun things together.
5. The way we respect each other's privacy.
6. The way we listen to each other.
7. The way we respect each other's belong ings.
8. The way we work out our problems.
9. The way we treat each other when we're mad or upset.
10. The way we do nice things for each other.

PARTICIPATION
PROCEDURE: The BLIND or LEADER SELECTION METHOD is used.

SUGGESTIONS: The leader may want to use more specific situations to get at the actual relationship issues. Support providers, families and special friends can be helpful in providing such information if group members are unable to do so.

TITLE: "We All Win"

SOCIALIZATION
GOAL AREA: Prosocial/Learning to Get Along With Others

MATERIALS: 3" × 5" "Problem Cards," "Winner" Cards for each member, Timer

GAME PROCEDURE: The leader tells members that in this game they will work together on problems so that everyone feels like a winner. Two members at a time take turns drawing a problem card and work together to find a solution that solves the problem for both of them within 30 seconds. Group members are asked to raise their winner cards if they think the solution will work. If not, members are asked to suggest a different solution that *will* work. The game continues until all cards have been used.

Problem scenarios include:

1. two persons both want to use the phone to call friends.
2. two persons want pop and there is only one can.
3. two persons want to go out to eat at different restaurants.
4. two persons want to watch different TV shows.
5. two persons want to talk to the boss at the same time.
6. two persons want to do something fun, but don't have any money.
7. two persons are living together, one wants to talk and the other wants private time.
8. two persons want to play different music on the radio.
9. two persons each like the same friend.
10. the dishes are dirty.
11. two persons both want to vacuum.
12. one gets to visit family or friends and the other doesn't.

PARTICIPATION
PROCEDURE: The BLIND or LEADER SELECTION METHOD is used.

TITLE: **"Doin' the Spring Thing"**

SOCIALIZATION
GOAL AREA: Prosocial/Learning to Get Along With Others

MATERIALS: Stimulus cards with spring related themes (words) listed on each card

GAME PROCEDURE: Group members take turns drawing theme cards and then choose a partner to act out the theme. Group members are then asked to guess the theme. Leaders and/or "actors" may give hints to help other members identify the theme. Members take turns until all theme cards have been drawn.

PARTICIPATION
PROCEDURE: The BLIND SELECTION METHOD is used.

SUGGESTIONS: Themes could include:

1. spring flowers growing
2. rain coming down
3. birds flying
4. sun shining
5. gardening
6. riding bikes
7. flying kites
8. taking walks
9. picnicking
10. baseball
11. fishing

SOCIAL COMPETENCE
(BEING A PART OF MY COMMUNITY)

"Being Responsible" I
"Being Responsible" II
"Don't Lose Your Cool" I
"Don't Lose Your Cool" II
"Mix and Match" I
"Weather Match"
"Should I Ask for Help?"
"Something's Wrong with Those Clothes!"
"The Greeting Game"
"Mix and Match" II
"Who Can Help?"
"Mix and Match" III
"Whose Problem?"
"Finding My Way"
"Thumbs Up or Thumbs Down" I
"Thumbs Up or Thumbs Down" II
"What Would You Do?"
"OK or No Way"
"You're The Boss"
"Stop and Think"
"What Works For Me When I'm Sad"
"What Works For Me When I'm Mad"
"Please Don't Tease" I
"Please Don't Tease" II
"Polite or Not Right"
"Would This Person Be A Good Friend?"

TITLE: **"Being Responsible" I**

SOCIALIZATION
GOAL AREA: Social Competence/Being A Part of My Community

MATERIALS: Responsibility Award certificates or facsimiles for each member

GAME PROCEDURE: Each member is given one of the certificates. The leader tells group members that people who are responsible (i.e. take care of themselves, their things, their jobs, etc.) sometimes receive special attention and awards. The leader then presents one situation at a time (enacts and/or verbalizes) to which members must decide whether the behavior was responsible or not. If the situation represents responsible behavior, members are instructed to hold up their certificates. If not, the certificate remains in their laps.

1. Individual doesn't do his chores.
2. Individual is tired and trades chores with someone else.
3. Individual is sick and doesn't go to work or call supervisor.
4. Individual is sick and calls work to tell them he/she won't be in.
5. Individual is sick, but doesn't want to tell anyone.
6. Individual is sick and asks for help or goes to the doctor.
7. Individual takes his/her friend's money from the table.
8. Individual asks to borrow a friend's shampoo.
9. Individual is upset with a friend so he hits him.

10. Individual is upset with a friend and talks to him about it.

11. Individual goes to work only when he feels like it.

12. Individual goes to work every day.

PARTICIPATION
PROCEDURE: All members participate at the same time.

TITLE: **"Being Responsible" II**

SOCIALIZATION
GOAL AREA: Social Competence/Being A Part of My Community

MATERIALS: Small box or container, slips of paper each listing a problem situation

GAME PROCEDURE: One member selects a problem slip from the container. The problem is read to the group. The member is asked to solve the problem in a responsible way. Other group members are encouraged to provide other ways of solving the problem.

Possible problems include:

1. Your neighbor was injured and can't get to her mailbox.

2. Someone left a bicycle in your yard.

3. You keep missing your bus to work.

4. You get some strange telephone calls about money.

5. You see that your neighbor's garbage cans have blown into the street.

6. You find a wallet on the floor in a store.

PARTICIPATION
PROCEDURE: The BLIND SELECTION METHOD is used.

SUGGESTIONS: The leader may want to ask members to share personal experiences related to responsible behavior. Topic areas include being responsible at work, at home, in the community, or with friends. Leaders are encouraged to make problems specific to the needs of the group.

TITLE:	**"Don't Lose Your Cool!" I**
SOCIALIZATION GOAL AREA:	Social Competence/Being A Part of My Community
MATERIALS:	No special materials are required
GAME PROCEDURE:	One member is selected to go to the center of the circle. The leader gives the member a situation, (changing for each individual), and asks the member what he/she would do. The group is prompted to respond to the center member. If he/she responds in a socially appropriate way, the group responds "He/she was cool"; if not, the response is "He/she lost his/her cool!"

Situations:

1. Someone asks you to put out your cigarette.
2. You can't find your keys.
3. Someone hit you for no reason.
4. You lost your money in the pop machine.
5. You want to see your supervisor right away.
6. You feel too sick to go to work.
7. You just don't want to go to work.
8. You're told to wait for coffee.
9. Someone gives you the finger or makes a fist.
10. Your class or work is cancelled.
11. Someone calls you a name.
12. At work, you're asked to do something you don't want to do.

PARTICIPATION PROCEDURE:	The BLIND or LEADER SELECTION METHOD may be used.

TITLE: **"Don't Lose Your Cool" II**

SOCIALIZATION
GOAL AREA: Social Competence/Being A Part of My Community

MATERIALS: No special materials are required

GAME PROCEDURE: One member is selected to participate with the leader in an enactment which shows either a "cool" or "uncool" way to respond to a particular situation. The group is prompted to respond to the situation with the proper rating e.g. "He/she was cool" or "He/she lost his/her cool."

Role enactments:

1. One member teases the other.
2. One member takes something from the other.
3. One member threatens the other with a gesture.
4. One member calls the other a name.
5. One member grabs the other.
6. One member talks without listening to the other.
7. One member bumps into the other.
8. Takes deep breaths and counts to 10.

Responses include:

1. Throw object.
2. Use names or foul language.
3. Walk away.
4. Tell person that you're not going to listen to them.
5. Tell person that you don't like that.
6. Stamp feet and tantrum.
7. Threaten to hit.

PARTICIPATION
PROCEDURE: The BLIND SELECTION METHOD is used.

SUGGESTIONS: The leader will initially want to participate as the responder to the incident while instructing the member as to his/her role. Nonverbal members may be encouraged to rate the response with a "thumbs-up" or "thumbs-down" gesture.

TITLE: **"Mix And Match" I**

SOCIALIZATION
GOAL AREA: Social Competence/Being A Part of My Community

MATERIALS: Magazine pictures or photographs depicting various clothing items

GAME PROCEDURE: One group member is selected to make an outfit from the pictures. The group judges whether the outfit is "OK" or "Not." When the outfit is judged as "OK," members applaud. If "Not," members are asked to suggest alternative choices.

PARTICIPATION
PROCEDURE: The BLIND SELECTION METHOD is used.

SUGGESTIONS: This game may be increased in difficulty level by requiring the member to "beat the clock" or perform task in _____ seconds. In addition, other clothing items, shoes, accessories, may be added to require a complete set of clothing. The leader may want to discuss personal styles/preferences or cultural/climate influences on style.

TITLE: **"Weather Match"**

SOCIALIZATION
GOAL AREA: Social Competence/Being A Part of My Community

MATERIALS: Cards depicting weather conditions: sun and swimming, rain and umbrella, snow and snowman. Photos or pictures of raincoat, hat, coat, sweater, boots, shorts, sandals

GAME PROCEDURE: One member selects a weather condition from the three stimulus cards: (1) hot and sunny, (2) rain, (3) snow and cold. Another member is selected to choose clothing cards/photos that match the weather. The group votes as to whether the clothing "matches" for the weather. If not, a member is selected by raised hands to assist. The procedure is continued until all members have had a turn.

PARTICIPATION
PROCEDURE: The BLIND SELECTION METHOD is used

SUGGESTIONS: Categories for matching could be expanded to include aspects of different cultures such as clothing, food, customs or other special practices.

TITLE: **"Should I Ask For Help?"**

SOCIALIZATION
GOAL AREA: Social Competence/Being A Part of My Community

MATERIALS: Container with slips of paper for each situation

GAME PROCEDURE: A member selects a situation from the problem box and must decide whether he/she needs help or can solve it on his/her own. Members are asked to respond with "I need help", or "I can do it myself." For less verbal members, "yes", or "no" or headshakes indicating "yes" or "no" would be appropriate.

Possible situations include:

1. You fell down, but aren't hurt.

2. You fell down and hurt your leg.

3. You haven't done your chores.

4. You don't know how to do a chore.

5. You can't find your money, but haven't looked.

6. Your money was stolen.

7. You need some shampoo or toothpaste.

8. The shampoo is all gone.

9. It's time to get ready for work.

10. You need some new clothes.

11. Your room or locker is a mess.

12. Something in your room is broken and needs to be fixed.

PARTICIPATION
PROCEDURE: The BLIND SELECTION METHOD is used.

TITLE: **"Something's Wrong With Those Clothes!"**

SOCIALIZATION
GOAL AREA: Social Competence/Being A Part of My Community

MATERIALS: Articles of clothing that need repair, e.g., broken zipper, missing buttons; articles that are too large; articles that don't match

GAME PROCEDURE: A member is selected to leave the area. The leader assists the member in putting on clothing or modifying his/her own clothing so that it is inappropriate. The person then enters the area and group members are asked to raise their hands when they recognize the problem with the person's clothing. One member is selected to go up, and point to what is inappropriate and to help the person fix the clothing.

Examples of modifications include:

1. Wearing a slightly torn shirt.
2. Rolling up pant legs.
3. Untying shoe laces.
4. Tucking pants into socks.
5. Putting a sweater on backwards.
6. Wearing socks that don't match.
7. Wearing a shirt missing a button.
8. Wearing a shirt that is buttoned wrong.
9. Wearing a sweater that is inside out.
10. Wearing shoes on the wrong feet.
11. Having underwear sticking out.

PARTICIPATION
PROCEDURE: The BLIND SELECTION METHOD is used to select one group member at a time.

SUGGESTIONS: This game can be modified to deal with idiosyncratic dressing behavior.

TITLE: **"The Greeting Game"**

SOCIALIZATION
GOAL AREA: Social Competence/Being A Part of My Community

MATERIALS: No special materials are required

GAME PROCEDURE: The leader role plays a "weird" greeting, e.g., hugging a person or pulling at a person, and then role plays an "OK" greeting (e.g., shaking hands or holding up hand and saying "Hi!"). After each role play the leader asks group members whether the scene was "weird" or "OK." The leader selects two group members to role play a greeting scene. Other group members can rate the role play scene as either "weird" or "OK." In order to encourage the group members who are role playing to use "OK" behavior, each person should have a chance to role play both "weird" and "OK" ways of greeting.

Suggestions for role play:

WEIRD

1. Hugging another person.
2. Kissing another person.
3. Pulling at a person's clothing.
4. Grabbing someone from behind.
5. Stroking or rubbing a person's back.
6. Holding hands.
7. Making direct face contact with someone.
8. Saying "Hey, honey."
9. Saying nothing.

OK

1. Shaking hands.
2. Holding up hand to wave.
3. Verbal phrases:
   a. "Hi!"
   b. "What's your name?"
   c. "My name is . . ."

The session should end by involving group members in "OK" role plays.

PARTICIPATION
PROCEDURE: The BLIND SELECTION PROCEDURE is used to select two group members at a time until all members have participated.

SUGGESTIONS: This game model may be used to address learning about social rules in various settings, i.e., appropriate table manners, locating restrooms, asking for help, dating, sexual activity.

TITLE: **"Mix and Match" II**

SOCIALIZATION
GOAL AREA: Social Competence/Being A Part of My Community

MATERIALS: Magazine pictures mounted on cards/paper or photographs of people in clothes that depict various types of dress. (i.e., party clothes, work clothes, exercise clothes, lounging clothes); box/container

GAME PROCEDURE: Group members take turns selecting a picture card and then tell the group an "OK" place or situation that matches the clothes. For example a member could say "I would wear these clothes to *a party.*" Group members are asked to respond as to whether they agree or have other ideas or suggestions.

PARTICIPATION PROCEDURE: The BLIND or LEADER SELECTION METHOD may be used.

SUGGESTIONS: If members are unable to respond, the leader may want to offer two or three choices. Leaders may also want to include pictures/photos of unusual or funny clothing for member's reactions.

TITLE: "Who Can Help?"

SOCIALIZATION GOAL AREA: Social Competence/Being A Part of My Community

MATERIALS: Index cards (or photos) with magazine pictures and titles of helpers such as policeman, fireman, support staff person, case manager, social worker, work supervisor, friend, counselor, etc.; box of containers with problem situations on slips of paper

GAME PROCEDURE: A member selects a problem situation from the "problem box" and then must pick the appropriate helper from the index cards.

Possible problems include:

1. You see smoke coming from your neighbor's house.
2. You are lost.
3. You don't know how to do your job.
4. You didn't get your SSI check.
5. Your wallet was stolen.
6. You lost your money.
7. You want to go to a movie with someone.
8. You want to learn how to take the bus.
9. You want a job.
10. You want to talk to someone.

PARTICIPATION
PROCEDURE: The BLIND SELECTION METHOD is used.

SUGGESTIONS: A leader may want to simplify the game by limiting the number of helpers to two or three specific to the accessibility of group members.

TITLE: **"Mix and Match" III**

SOCIALIZATION
GOAL AREA: Social Competence/Being A Part of My Community

MATERIALS: (1) magazine pictures, sketches, written descriptions of situations suggested below; (2) photos or pictures of clothing that goes with situations suggested below

GAME PROCEDURE: A group member selects one of the stimulus cards and identifies the situation. The member then chooses the clothing picture appropriate to the situation depicted on the card. Group members vote "OK" or "NOT" with respect to the appropriateness of the clothing.

Possible situations include:

1. Dinner Party	6. Concert
2. Work	7. Costume Party
3. School	8. Nighttime
4. Beach	9. Jogging/Walking
5. Picnic	

PARTICIPATION PROCEDURE: The BLIND SELECTION METHOD is used.

SUGGESTIONS: The game may be modified by having other group members, (1) select another appropriate match; or (2) describe personal clothing preferences.

TITLE: "Whose Problem?"

SOCIALIZATION GOAL AREA: Social Competence (work)/Being A Part of My Community

MATERIALS: No specific materials needed

GAME PROCEDURE: The group leader takes turns giving group members scenarios to determine *who* has the problem, by indicating "my problem" or "someone else's problem." Situations could include:

1. Co-worker is upset about his job.
2. Two other co-workers argue about their job.
3. Co-worker tells you "You are not doing your job right."
4. Supervisor is upset about you coming to work late.
5. Supervisor and co-worker are arguing about the job.
6. You and a co-worker get in trouble for talking instead of working.
7. Co-worker tells you to take a longer break and you get in trouble with your supervisor.
8. You forgot to bring your lunch to work.

PARTICIPATION
PROCEDURE: The LEADER SELECTION or BLIND SELECTION METHOD is used.

TITLE: **"Finding My Way"**

SOCIALIZATION
GOAL AREA: Social Competence/Being A Part of My Community

MATERIALS: No specific materials needed

GAME PROCEDURE: Members take turns assuming the role of an individual who is lost in the community. The leader presents possible solutions and the member must determine whether it's an "OK" or "safe" way to find his/her way home. Members are encouraged to evaluate why certain solutions aren't safe or workable.

Suggested situations:

1. Just keep walking until you see your home.
2. Tell a bus driver where you live and ask how to get there.
3. Ask someone you don't know to drive you home.
4. Call your home and tell them you're lost.
5. Show your I.D. card to a policeman.
6. Sit down in the grass until someone finds you.
7. Walk into someone's house and tell them you're lost.
8. Go to a bank or store to find someone to help you.
9. Get on any bus you see.

PARTICIPATION
PROCEDURE: The BLIND or LEADER SELECTION METHOD is used.

TITLE: "Thumbs Up Or Thumbs Down" I

SOCIALIZATION
GOAL AREA: Social Competence (work)/Being A Part of
              My Community

MATERIALS: None

GAME PROCEDURE: The leader takes turns reading the scenarios
                   to group members and asks them to signal
                   "thumbs up or thumbs down." Members are
                   encouraged to explain their reasons and dis-
                   cuss any differences of opinion.

1. You come to work late because you were
   too tired to get up.
2. You miss your bus and call your boss to
   say you'll be late.
3. You wear the same clothes for two days
   in a row.
4. You come to work neat and clean.
5. You do your work the way you want to
   and not the way your boss told you.
6. You do what your boss tells you to do.
7. You take work materials home because
   you need them.
8. You leave work and go home when someone upsets you.
9. You go to your supervisor when you're
   having a problem.
10. You . . .

PARTICIPATION
PROCEDURE: Everyone has a chance to participate at the
              same time.

TITLE: "Thumbs Up Or Thumbs Down" II

SOCIALIZATION
GOAL AREA: Social Competence (work)/Being A Part of
              My Community

MATERIALS: None

GAME PROCEDURE: The leader takes turns reading the scenarios to group members and asks them to signal "thumbs up or thumbs down." Members are encouraged to explain their reasons and discuss any differences of opinion.

1. You tell your boss that you are having your period.
2. You hug a co-worker.
3. You talk about a work problem to your boss.
4. You ask a co-worker to eat lunch with you.
5. You tell your boss about your family's money problems.
6. You tell your boss about your money problem and ask for a raise.
7. You ask a co-worker for a date.
8. You walk away from your boss when he tells you about a mistake.
9. You listen to your boss and tell him you'll do better next time.
10. You follow a good-looking co-worker to get his/her attention.
11. You tell your boss about a co-worker's mistake.
12. You blame your co-workers for your mistakes.

PARTICIPATION
PROCEDURE: Everyone has a chance to participate at the same time.

TITLE: **"What Would You Do?"**

SOCIALIZATION
GOAL AREA: Social Competence (work)/Being A Part of My Community

MATERIALS: None

GAME PROCEDURE: The leader reads each scenario and asks the members to signal (raise hand, nod, press clicker, etc.) if the situation has happened to them. The leader then asks for a volunteer to tell what he/she did or would do in the situation.

1. Boss tells you that you made a mistake.
2. Boss tells you to stop what you're doing and change jobs.
3. Boss tells you co-workers have complained that you are bothering them.
4. Boss tells you to work faster.
5. Boss tells you that your work area is messy.
6. Boss tells you that you must get along with co-workers.
7. A co-worker makes fun of you.
8. A co-worker asks to borrow money from you.
9. A co-worker wants to talk to you while you are trying to work.
10. A co-worker keeps telling you what to do or how to do your work.
11. A co-worker threatens to hurt you.

PARTICIPATION
PROCEDURE: The LEADER SELECTION METHOD is used.

TITLE: **"OK Or No Way"**

SOCIALIZATION
GOAL AREA: Social Competence (work)/Being A Part of My Community

MATERIALS: Index cards depicting each scenario

GAME PROCEDURE: Leaders role play or ask members to assist with role plays of worker behavior on the job.

Group members are asked to rate each worker's response with "OK" or "No Way." For "No Way" responses, members are asked to replay the role of the worker and demonstrate an "OK" response. Other group members may be encouraged to demonstrate variations.

PARTICIPATION
PROCEDURE: Everyone in the group has a chance to participate at the same time.

SUGGESTIONS: Scenarios may be individualized, but could include:

In response to constructive criticism from Supervisor . . .

1. Worker walks away.
2. Worker listens and agrees to try to do better.
3. Worker complains that he/she doesn't like boss picking on him/her.
4. Worker blames co-worker.
5. Worker apologizes.
6. Worker loudly announces that he/she will quit.
7. Worker thanks boss for helping him/her.

TITLE: **"You're The Boss"**

SOCIALIZATION
GOAL AREA: Social Competence/Being A Part of My Community

MATERIALS: 3″ × 5″ cards listing each scenario. Cards are turned upside down and placed in a container.

GAME PROCEDURE: Members take turns choosing a card and responding to the situation as the "boss." The leader asks the "boss" how the situation causes a problem at work and what the "boss" wants the worker to change to be a better worker.

Other members are encouraged to agree or disagree.

1. Worker comes to work one hour late.
2. Worker doesn't come to work and doesn't call.
3. Worker breaks something and hides it from you.
4. Worker comes to work and smells bad.
5. Worker curses at co-workers when upset.
6. Worker tells you a lie about a co-worker.
7. Worker doesn't do what you tell him/her to do.
8. Worker is asleep at work.
9. Worker steals money from your desk.
10. Worker talks back to you.

PARTICIPATION
PROCEDURE: The BLIND or LEADER SELECTION METHOD is used.

TITLE: **"Stop And Think"**

SOCIALIZATION
GOAL AREA: Social Competence (work)/Being A Part of My Community

MATERIALS: 3″ × 5″ index cards with the messages below

GAME PROCEDURE: Leader reads index cards to group members. Members will use thumbs up or thumbs down in response to different messages or topics. Examples can include:

1. Do I tell my boss private things about my boyfriend/girlfriend?
2. Do I tell my co-worker about my money?
3. Do I tell my supervisor "Leave me alone?"
4. Do I tell my supervisor if I'm not feeling well?

5. Do I tell my supervisor what I want to buy for myself or a friend?

6. Do I tell my supervisor if I need help with work?

7. Do I call my supervisor "Sweetie Pie" or "Hey Babe?"

PARTICIPATION
PROCEDURE: Everyone has a chance to participate at the same time.

TITLE: **"What Works For Me When I'm Sad"**

SOCIALIZATION
GOAL AREA: Social Competence/Being A Part of My Community

MATERIALS: Index cards that have individual coping responses listed

GAME PROCEDURE: The leader tells group members that the game focuses on different ways that help people feel better when they are sad. Members take turns drawing "coping cards" and responding with "this works for me" or "this doesn't work for me." Other group members are then encouraged to signal in response to "this works or doesn't work for me."

PARTICIPATION
PROCEDURE: BLIND or LEADER SELECTION METHOD is used.

SUGGESTIONS: Suggested coping responses include:

1. Talk to a friend.
2. Listen to music.
3. Find something fun to do.
4. Talk to my counselor.
5. Take a bath.
6. Take a walk.
7. Go to a movie.

8. Go out to dinner with a friend.
9. Stay alone.
10. Talk to my family.
11. Go shopping.
12. Eat everything in the refrigerator.
13. Smoke a cigarette.

TITLE:	**"What Works for Me When I'm Mad"**
SOCIALIZATION GOAL AREA:	Social Competence/Being A Part of My Community
MATERIALS:	Index cards that have individual coping responses listed
GAME PROCEDURE:	The leader tells group members that the game focuses on different ways that help people feel better when they are mad. Members take turns drawing "coping cards" and responding with "this works for me" or "this doesn't work for me." Other group members are then encouraged to signal in response to this works or doesn't work for me.
PARTICIPATION PROCEDURE:	BLIND or LEADER SELECTION METHOD is used.
SUGGESTIONS:	Suggested coping responses include:

1. Saying how I feel.
2. Walking away/taking a walk.
3. Talking to someone.
4. Listening to music.
5. Ignoring.
6. Telling people to "leave me alone."
7. Going to my room.
8. Writing down my feelings.

9. Working out a problem.
10. Talking to my counselor.
11. Doing exercises.
12. Squeezing a ball/pillow.

TITLE: **"Please Don't Tease" I**

SOCIALIZATION
GOAL AREA: Social Competence/Being A Part of My Community

MATERIALS: Construction paper, stop signs attached to popsicle sticks/or tongue depressors or stop signs drawn on index cards

GAME PROCEDURE: The leader hands out stop signs to each member and tells them that they are to hold up the sign to signal that a particular teasing behavior is hurtful and needs to stop. The leader proceeds to enact different types of teasing. Group members will be encouraged to discriminate between friendly and hurtful types of teasing.

Possible demonstrations include:

1. Making funny faces.
2. Repeating words or actions.
3. Two fingers held behind a person's head.
4. Making threatening gestures (i.e., fist pounding).
5. Making fun of how a person looks.
6. Making fun of what a person is wearing.
7. Telling a person that he/she is stupid.
8. Name rhyming (Barb, farb; Tom, mom).
9. Making fun of mannerisms (i.e., the way a person walks or talks).

PARTICIPATION
PROCEDURE: All members participate at the same time.

TITLE: **"Please Don't Tease" II**

SOCIALIZATION
GOAL AREA: Social Competence/Being A Part of My Community

MATERIALS: Construction paper, stop signs attached to popsicle sticks/or tongue depressors, or stop signs drawn on index cards

GAME PROCEDURE: The leader hands out stop signs to each member and tells them that they are to hold up the sign to signal that a particular response to teasing needs to stop. If the response to teasing is OK, members are to leave their signs down. For responses that need to stop, members will be encouraged to demonstrate a better way to respond.

Sample scenarios could include:

1. In response to teasing, the person cries and puts his/her head down.
2. In response to teasing, the person says "please don't tease."
3. In response to teasing, the person walks away.
4. In response to teasing, the person stomps his/her feet and throws something.
5. In response to teasing, the person teases back.
6. In response to teasing, the person laughs.
7. In response to teasing, the person asks the teaser to stop and then reports to support person.
8. In response to teasing, the person calls 911.
9. In response to teasing, the person screams and yells.

PARTICIPATION
PROCEDURE: All members participate at the same time.

TITLE: **"Polite Or Not Right"**

SOCIALIZATION
GOAL AREA: Social Competence/Being A Part of My Community

MATERIALS: Index cards with statements or scenarios individually written

GAME PROCEDURE: The leader tells members that the game will focus on behaviors or actions that are "polite" ways to treat others or "not right" ways to treat others. Members will take turns drawing cards and the leader or group member (if able) will read the card and respond with "polite" or "not right." The remaining group members will then be asked to vote if they agree or disagree. For situations that are determined to be "not right," members will be asked to replay or correct the situation to make it right.

Sample situations could include:

1. "Give me that book."
2. "Please don't talk to me when I'm working/ busy."
3. "Stop looking at me."
4. "I should not have yelled at you."
5. Individual interrupts supervisor/teacher.
6. Individual bumps into another person and says nothing.
7. Individual shares pop with a friend and friend says nothing.
8. Individual receives a gift and walks away.
9. Individual says, "Excuse me, but the phone is for you."
10. Individual says, "Thank you for helping me with that problem."

PARTICIPATION
PROCEDURE: The BLIND or LEADER SELECTION METHOD is used

SUGGESTIONS: The sample situations or scenarios could be modified to make them more relevant to the specific social context (i.e., work, school, family, home).

TITLE: **"Would This Person Be A Good Friend?"**

SOCIALIZATION
GOAL AREA: Social Competence/Being A Part of My Community

MATERIALS: 3″ × 5″ Index cards that depict a "thumbs up" or "smiling face" on one side and a scenario on the other side

GAME PROCEDURE: The leader presents the cards to group members. Each member draws one card. The leader then selects one member to begin by reading the scenario. The member is asked to hold up his/her card if the scenario describes a "good friend" or keep it down, if not. All other members are then asked to respond in the same manner. Members take turns until all have had a turn.

GAME PROCEDURE:
1. Person asks you to steal for them.
2. Person asks you again and again for money/cigarettes and never pays you back.
3. Person shares pizza with you.
4. Person borrows $1.00 and pays you back.
5. Person tries to kiss your boyfriend/girlfriend.
6. Person threatens to hurt you.
7. Person helps you when you're not feeling well.
8. Person makes or buys you a cup of coffee.
9. Person asks you to go out to eat.
10. Person gets in your wallet and takes your money.

PARTICIPATION
PROCEDURE: The LEADER or BLIND SELECTION METHOD is used.

BIBLIOGRAPHY

Bendekovic, John. *Working with a Group.* Washington: The United States Justice Department (Grant #1491-00-F1-71), 1971.

Edmonson, Barbara; Moxley, David; & Nevil, Nevalyn. Continued Development and Demonstration of a Program for Disturbed Retarded Institutional Residents. Final report of service development project FY 79 #00474, Ohio Department of Mental health and Mental Retardation, Division of Mental Retardation and Developmental Disabilities, Columbus, Ohio: The Nisonger Center, The Ohio State University, 1980.

Edmonson, Barbara; Nevil, Nevalyn; & Moxley, David. "Developing Responsible Self Directed Behavior." 27-minute videotape cassette. Columbus, Ohio: The Nisonger Center, The Ohio State University, 1980.

Han, Sung Soon. Use of Socialization Games to Increase Prosocial Behavior of Institutionalized Retarded Women. Unpublished doctoral dissertation. The Ohio State University, 1980.

Moxley, David; Nevil, Nevalyn; & Edmonson, Barbara. "Meeting Time: Structured Group Activities with the Mentally Retarded." 27-minute videotape cassette. Columbus, Ohio: The Nisonger Center, The Ohio State University, 1980.

Nevil, Nevalyn & Edmonson, Barbara. "A Visit to a Group Home." 7-minute synchronized sound 35 mm slide show. Columbus, Ohio: The Nisonger Center, The Ohio State University, 1980.

Rosen, Marvin; Clark, Gerald R.; & Kivitz, Marvin S. *Habilitation of the Handicapped.* Baltimore: University Park Press, 1977.

Rosen, Marvin & Hoffman, M. *Personal Adjustment Training,* Vol. III. *Appropriate Behavior Training: A Group Counseling Manual for the Mentally Handicapped.* Elwyn, Pennsylvania: The Elwyn Institute, 1975.

Schaefer, Charles E. & Reid, Steven E. (Ed): *Game Play.* New York, John Wiley & Sons, Inc., 1986.

Shapiro, Lawrence E. (Ed.): *The Book of Psychotherapeutic Games.* King of Prussia, The Center for Applied Psychology, Inc., 1993.

INDEX